THE AYURVEDA WAY

Transforming Your Life with Ancient Wisdom

Mei Lin Zhang

Table of Contents

- A New Zealand Made Product

Get A Free Book At: xspurts.com/posts/free-book-offer[4]

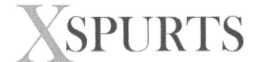

5

---

1. https://Xspurts.com

2. https://Xspurts.com

3. https://Xspurts.com

4. https://xspurts.com/posts/free-book-offer

5. https://xspurts.com/

Introduction to Ayurveda

Ayurveda is an ancient system of medicine that has been practiced in India for thousands of years. It is a holistic system of medicine that is focused on promoting health and wellness by balancing the body, mind, and spirit. Ayurveda is a Sanskrit word that means "knowledge of life" or "science of life".

According to Ayurvedic philosophy, health is not just the absence of disease but a state of balance between the three doshas, which are Vata, Pitta, and Kapha. Each individual has a unique combination of these doshas, and an imbalance in any of them can lead to illness.

The Vata dosha is associated with movement and is responsible for bodily functions such as breathing, circulation, and nerve impulses. Pitta is associated with digestion and metabolism and is responsible for maintaining the body's internal balance. Kapha is associated with structure and stability and is responsible for maintaining the body's physical and emotional stability.

1. Ayurveda believes that there are five elements that make up the universe and everything in it: earth, water, fire, air, and ether. These elements combine in various proportions to form the three doshas. Vata is composed of air and ether, Pitta is composed of fire and water, and Kapha is composed of earth and water.

Ayurvedic treatments are aimed at restoring balance to the doshas and the elements that make them up. Treatments may include dietary changes, herbal remedies, massage, yoga, meditation, and other practices.

One of the most well-known Ayurvedic practices is the use of herbal remedies. Ayurvedic practitioners use a wide variety of herbs to treat a range of ailments. Some of the most commonly used herbs in Ayurveda include ashwagandha, turmeric, ginger, and holy basil.

Another key component of Ayurveda is diet. Ayurvedic practitioners believe that food is medicine and that a balanced diet is essential for good health. Foods are categorized according to their taste, and each taste is associated with a particular dosha. For example, sweet foods are associated with Kapha, sour foods are associated with Pitta, and bitter and astringent foods are associated with Vata.

Ayurveda also places a great emphasis on daily routines and self-care practices. Ayurvedic practitioners believe that daily routines and self-care practices, such as oil massage and meditation, are essential for maintaining good health and preventing illness.

Yoga and meditation are also important components of Ayurveda. Ayurvedic practitioners believe that yoga and meditation help to balance the doshas and promote good health. Yoga is a physical practice that is designed to improve flexibility, strength, and balance. Meditation is a mental practice that is designed to calm the mind and promote inner peace.

Ayurveda has been used to treat a wide variety of ailments, from minor illnesses to chronic conditions. Ayurvedic practitioners believe that by treating the whole person, not just the symptoms of a particular ailment, they can help to promote good health and prevent future illness.

In recent years, Ayurveda has become increasingly popular in the West, as more and more people are seeking out natural and holistic approaches to healthcare. While there is still much debate about the effectiveness of Ayurveda, many people have found relief from a wide variety of conditions through Ayurvedic treatments.

The origins and history of Ayurveda

Ayurveda is an ancient system of medicine that has been practiced in India for thousands of years. Its origins can be traced back to the Vedas, which are the ancient texts of Hinduism. Ayurveda is believed to have been developed by the sages and seers of ancient India who lived thousands of years ago.

The origins of Ayurveda can be traced back to the Vedic period, which is believed to have started around 3000 BCE. During this time, the sages and seers of ancient India were studying the human body and its relationship to nature. They observed the plants and animals around them and noticed how they responded to different environmental factors.

It is believed that the knowledge of Ayurveda was passed down orally from one generation to another until it was eventually written down in the form of the Ayurvedic texts. The most important of these texts are the Charaka Samhita, the Sushruta Samhita, and the Ashtanga Hridaya.

The Charaka Samhita is one of the oldest and most important Ayurvedic texts. It is believed to have been written around 1500 BCE and is attributed to the sage Charaka. The text is divided into eight sections, each of which covers a different aspect of Ayurveda. The Charaka Samhita covers topics such as diagnosis, treatment, and prevention of disease.

The Sushruta Samhita is another important Ayurvedic text. It is believed to have been written around 600 BCE and is attributed to the sage Sushruta. The text is divided into six sections, each of which covers a different aspect of Ayurveda. The Sushruta Samhita covers topics such as surgery, ophthalmology, and obstetrics.

The Ashtanga Hridaya is a more recent Ayurvedic text. It was written in the 7th century CE and is attributed to the sage Vagbhata. The text is divided into six sections, each of which covers a different aspect of Ayurveda. The Ashtanga Hridaya covers topics such as diagnosis, treatment, and prevention of disease.

Ayurveda was also influenced influenced by other ancient medical systems, such as the Greek and Roman systems. The Greek physician Hippocrates, who is considered the father of Western medicine, is believed to have been influenced by Ayurvedic principles.

During the medieval period, Ayurveda continued to develop and evolve. Many new texts were written, and the knowledge of Ayurveda was passed down through the generations. Ayurveda was also influenced by other ancient medical systems, such as the Chinese system of medicine.

In the 18th and 19th centuries, Ayurveda faced challenges from the British colonial government, which was suspicious of traditional Indian medical systems. The British introduced their own system of medicine, which was based on Western medical principles. Ayurveda was marginalized and faced many challenges during this period.

In the early 20th century, there was a resurgence of interest in Ayurveda, as Indians began to question the validity of Western medical systems. Ayurveda was recognized by the Indian government as a legitimate system of medicine, and efforts were made to promote and develop Ayurveda.

Today, Ayurveda is recognized as a legitimate system of medicine in India, and it is practiced by millions of people around the world. Ayurvedic treatments are increasingly being used to complement Western medical treatments, and many people are turning to Ayurveda for its holistic approach to healthcare.

The guiding principles of Ayurveda

Ayurveda is an ancient system of medicine that has been practiced in India for thousands of years. It is a holistic system of medicine that is focused on promoting health and wellness by balancing the body, mind, and spirit. The guiding principles of Ayurveda are based on the belief that the body and mind are interconnected and that a balance between the two is essential for good health.

The first guiding principle of Ayurveda is the belief that each individual is unique. Ayurveda recognizes that each person has a unique physical and mental constitution, and that what may work for one person may not work for another. Therefore, Ayurveda takes a personalized approach to healthcare, with treatments tailored to each individual's needs.

The second guiding principle of Ayurveda is the belief in the three doshas. As mentioned earlier, the three doshas are Vata, Pitta, and Kapha. Each dosha is associated with different physical and mental characteristics, and an imbalance in any of the doshas can lead to illness. Ayurvedic treatments are aimed at restoring balance to the doshas.

The third guiding principle of Ayurveda is the belief in the five elements. Ayurveda recognizes that everything in the universe is made up of five elements - earth, water, fire, air, and ether. These elements combine in different ways to form the doshas, and an imbalance in any of the elements can lead to illness. Ayurvedic treatments are aimed at restoring balance to the elements.

The fourth guiding principle of Ayurveda is the belief in the importance of digestion. Ayurveda recognizes that digestion is essential for good health, and that poor digestion can lead to illness. Therefore, Ayurveda places a great emphasis on maintaining a healthy digestive system through diet and lifestyle.

The fifth guiding principle of Ayurveda is the belief in the importance of daily routines and self-care practices. Ayurveda recognizes that daily routines and self-care practices, such as oil massage and meditation, are essential for maintaining good health and preventing illness.

The sixth guiding principle of Ayurveda is the belief in the importance of a balanced diet. Ayurveda recognizes that food is medicine and that a balanced diet is essential for good health. Foods are categorized according to their taste, and each taste is associated with a particular dosha. For example, sweet foods are associated with Kapha, sour foods are associated with Pitta, and bitter and astringent foods are associated with Vata.

The seventh guiding principle of Ayurveda is the belief in the importance of herbal remedies. Ayurvedic practitioners use a wide variety of herbs to treat a range of ailments. Some of the most commonly used herbs in Ayurveda include ashwagandha, turmeric, ginger, and holy basil.

The eighth guiding principle of Ayurveda is the belief in the importance of yoga and meditation. Ayurvedic practitioners believe that yoga and meditation help to balance the doshas and promote good health. Yoga is a physical practice that is designed to improve flexibility, strength, and balance. Meditation is a mental practice that is designed to calm the mind and promote inner peace.

Understanding the five elements and the three doshas

Ayurveda is an ancient system of medicine that is focused on promoting health and wellness by balancing the body, mind, and spirit. Ayurveda recognizes that everything in the universe is made up of five elements - earth, water, fire, air, and ether. These elements combine in different ways to form the three doshas - Vata, Pitta, and Kapha. Understanding the five elements and the three doshas is key to understanding Ayurvedic principles and treatments.

The five elements that make up the universe are earth, water, fire, air, and ether. These elements are believed to combine in different ways to form everything in the universe, including the human body. Each element is associated with different qualities and characteristics.

Earth is associated with stability, structure, and heaviness. Water is associated with fluidity, cohesion, and coolness. Fire is associated with heat, transformation, and energy. Air is associated with movement, lightness, and dryness. Ether is associated with space, emptiness, and sound.

The three doshas - Vata, Pitta, and Kapha - are believed to be made up of different combinations of these elements. Each dosha is associated with different physical and mental characteristics, and an imbalance in any of the doshas can lead to illness.

Vata is composed of air and ether. It is associated with movement and is responsible for bodily functions such as breathing, circulation, and nerve impulses. When Vata is in balance, a person is energetic, creative, and adaptable. When Vata is out of balance, a person may experience anxiety, insomnia, and digestive issues.

Pitta is composed of fire and water. It is associated with digestion and metabolism and is responsible for maintaining the body's internal balance. When Pitta is in balance, a person is intelligent, focused, and ambitious. When Pitta is out of balance, a person may experience anger, inflammation, and skin issues.

Kapha is composed of earth and water. It is associated with structure and stability and is responsible for maintaining the body's physical and emotional stability. When Kapha is in balance, a person is calm, loving, and nurturing. When Kapha is out of balance, a person may experience lethargy, weight gain, and respiratory issues.

Ayurvedic treatments are aimed at restoring balance to the doshas and the elements that make them up. Treatments may include dietary changes, herbal remedies, massage, yoga, meditation, and other practices. For example, if a person has an imbalance in Vata, they may be advised to eat warm, nourishing foods, practice grounding yoga poses, and use warming herbs such as ginger and cinnamon.

Understanding the five elements and the three doshas is key to understanding Ayurvedic principles and treatments. Ayurveda recognizes that each individual is unique and that what may work for one person may not work for another. Therefore, Ayurveda takes a personalized approach to healthcare, with treatments tailored to each individual's needs.

The Three Doshas: Vata, Pitta, and Kapha

1. Ayurveda is an ancient system of medicine that is focused on promoting health and wellness by balancing the body, mind, and spirit. Ayurveda recognizes that each person has a unique physical and mental constitution, and that what may work for one person may not work for another. Ayurveda categorizes these unique constitutions into three doshas: Vata, Pitta, and Kapha. Understanding the three doshas is key to understanding Ayurvedic principles and treatments.

Vata is composed of air and ether, and it is responsible for bodily functions such as breathing, circulation, and nerve impulses. Vata is associated with movement and change and is responsible for the movements of the body's organs and tissues. People with a Vata constitution tend to be thin, have dry skin and hair, and have a tendency to feel cold. They are often creative, enthusiastic, and have a quick mind. When Vata is out of balance, however, people may experience anxiety, nervousness, insomnia, and digestive issues.

Pitta is composed of fire and water, and it is responsible for digestion and metabolism. Pitta is associated with heat and energy and is responsible for the body's internal balance. People with a Pitta constitution tend to have a medium build, oily skin and hair, and a tendency to feel hot. They are often intelligent, ambitious, and confident. When Pitta is out of balance, however, people may experience anger, inflammation, and skin issues.

Kapha is composed of earth and water, and it is responsible for the body's structure and stability. Kapha is associated with stability and endurance and is responsible for maintaining the body's physical and emotional stability. People with a Kapha constitution tend to have a heavier build, soft skin and hair, and a tendency to feel cold. They are often calm, loving, and nurturing. When Kapha is out of balance, however, people may experience lethargy, weight gain, and respiratory issues.

Ayurvedic treatments are aimed at restoring balance to the doshas and the elements that make them up. Treatments may include dietary changes, herbal remedies, massage, yoga, meditation, and other practices. For example, if a person has an imbalance in Pitta, they may be advised to eat cooling foods, practice calming yoga poses, and use cooling herbs such as coriander and fennel.

It is important to note that each person has a unique combination of the three doshas, and no two people are exactly the same. Additionally, each person's doshic balance can change over time, depending on factors such as diet, lifestyle, and environmental factors. Ayurveda recognizes this and takes a personalized approach to healthcare, with treatments tailored to each individual's needs.

Understanding the three doshas is key to understanding Ayurvedic principles and treatments. Ayurveda recognizes that each person is unique and that what may work for one person may not work for another. Therefore, Ayurveda takes a personalized approach to healthcare, with treatments tailored to each individual's needs. By understanding your unique doshic balance, you can make informed decisions about your health and wellness and take steps to restore balance when necessary.

Vata: The principle of movement

Vata is one of the three doshas in Ayurveda, along with Pitta and Kapha. Vata is composed of air and ether, and it is responsible for bodily functions such as breathing, circulation, and nerve impulses. Vata is associated with movement and change and is responsible for the movements of the body's organs and tissues. Understanding Vata is key to understanding Ayurvedic principles and treatments.

People with a Vata constitution tend to be thin, have dry skin and hair, and have a tendency to feel cold. They are often creative, enthusiastic, and have a quick mind. When Vata is out of balance, however, people may experience anxiety, nervousness, insomnia, and digestive issues.

Ayurvedic treatments for Vata imbalances are aimed at restoring balance to the dosha and may include dietary changes, herbal remedies, massage, yoga, meditation, and other practices. For example, if a person has an imbalance in Vata, they may be advised to eat warm, nourishing foods, practice grounding yoga poses, and use warming herbs such as ginger and cinnamon.

Ayurveda recognizes that Vata is responsible for many of the body's movements, including the movements of the organs and tissues. Vata governs the body's movements by regulating the nervous system and controlling the flow of energy in the body. Vata is also responsible for the movement of thoughts and emotions.

Vata is important for maintaining the body's health and vitality, but an imbalance in Vata can lead to a range of health issues. When Vata is out of balance, people may experience anxiety, nervousness, insomnia, and digestive issues. Vata imbalances can also lead to dry skin, constipation, and joint pain.

Ayurvedic treatments for Vata imbalances are aimed at restoring balance to the dosha and may include dietary changes, herbal remedies, massage, yoga, meditation, and other practices. For example, if a person has an imbalance in Vata, they may be advised to eat warm, nourishing foods, practice grounding yoga poses, and use warming herbs such as ginger and cinnamon.

In addition to dietary changes and herbal remedies, massage is a popular Ayurvedic treatment for Vata imbalances. Ayurvedic massage, also known as abhyanga, involves the application of warm oil to the body. The warm oil helps to calm the nervous system and nourish the skin, while the massage itself helps to stimulate the flow of energy in the body and promote relaxation.

Yoga and meditation are also important Ayurvedic treatments for Vata imbalances. Yoga poses that are grounding and stabilizing, such as the mountain pose and the child's pose, can help to calm the nervous system and promote relaxation. Meditation is also effective for balancing Vata, as it helps to calm the mind and promote inner peace.

Pitta: The principle of transformation

Pitta is one of the three doshas in Ayurveda, along with Vata and Kapha. Pitta is composed of fire and water, and it is responsible for digestion and metabolism. Pitta is associated with heat and energy and is responsible for the body's internal balance. Understanding Pitta is key to understanding Ayurvedic principles and treatments.

People with a Pitta constitution tend to have a medium build, oily skin and hair, and a tendency to feel hot. They are often intelligent, ambitious, and confident. When Pitta is out of balance, however, people may experience anger, inflammation, and skin issues.

Ayurvedic treatments for Pitta imbalances are aimed at restoring balance to the dosha and may include dietary changes, herbal remedies, massage, yoga, meditation, and other practices. For example, if a person has an imbalance in Pitta, they may be advised to eat cooling foods, practice calming yoga poses, and use cooling herbs such as coriander and fennel.

Ayurveda recognizes that Pitta is responsible for digestion and metabolism. Pitta governs the body's metabolism by regulating the digestive system and controlling the flow of energy in the body. Pitta is also responsible for the transformation of emotions and experiences.

Pitta is important for maintaining the body's health and vitality, but an imbalance in Pitta can lead to a range of health issues. When Pitta is out of balance, people may experience anger, inflammation, and skin issues. Pitta imbalances can also lead to digestive issues, such as heartburn and acid reflux.

Ayurvedic treatments for Pitta imbalances are aimed at restoring balance to the dosha and may include dietary changes, herbal remedies, massage, yoga, meditation, and other practices. For example, if a person has an imbalance in Pitta, they may be advised to eat cooling foods, practice calming yoga poses, and use cooling herbs such as coriander and fennel.

In addition to dietary changes and herbal remedies, massage is a popular Ayurvedic treatment for Pitta imbalances. Ayurvedic massage, also known as abhyanga, involves the application of warm oil to the body. The warm oil helps to nourish the skin and calm the nervous system, while the massage itself helps to stimulate the flow of energy in the body and promote relaxation.

Yoga and meditation are also important Ayurvedic treatments for Pitta imbalances. Yoga poses that are cooling and calming, such as the moon salutation and the seated forward bend, can help to balance Pitta and promote relaxation. Meditation is also effective for balancing Pitta, as it helps to calm the mind and promote inner peace.

Kapha: The principle of structure and stability

Kapha is one of the three doshas in Ayurveda, along with Vata and Pitta. Kapha is composed of earth and water, and it is responsible for the body's structure and stability. Kapha is associated with stability and endurance and is responsible for maintaining the body's physical and emotional stability. Understanding Kapha is key to understanding Ayurvedic principles and treatments.

People with a Kapha constitution tend to have a heavier build, soft skin and hair, and a tendency to feel cold. They are often calm, loving, and nurturing. When Kapha is out of balance, however, people may experience lethargy, weight gain, and respiratory issues.

Ayurvedic treatments for Kapha imbalances are aimed at restoring balance to the dosha and may include dietary changes, herbal remedies, massage, yoga, meditation, and other practices. For example, if a person has an imbalance in Kapha, they may be advised to eat light, warming foods, practice invigorating yoga poses, and use stimulating herbs such as ginger and black pepper.

Ayurveda recognizes that Kapha is responsible for the body's structure and stability. Kapha governs the body's structure by regulating the skeletal system and controlling the flow of energy in the body. Kapha is also responsible for emotional stability and endurance.

Kapha is important for maintaining the body's health and vitality, but an imbalance in Kapha can lead to a range of health issues. When Kapha is out of balance, people may experience lethargy, weight gain, and respiratory issues. Kapha imbalances can also lead to depression and a lack of motivation.

Ayurvedic treatments for Kapha imbalances are aimed at restoring balance to the dosha and may include dietary changes, herbal remedies, massage, yoga, meditation, and other practices. For example, if a person has an imbalance in Kapha, they may be advised to eat light, warming foods, practice invigorating yoga poses, and use stimulating herbs such as ginger and black pepper.

In addition to dietary changes and herbal remedies, massage is a popular Ayurvedic treatment for Kapha imbalances. Ayurvedic massage, also known as abhyanga, involves the application of warm oil to the body. The warm oil helps to stimulate the flow of energy in the body and promote relaxation.

Yoga and meditation are also important Ayurvedic treatments for Kapha imbalances. Yoga poses that are invigorating and stimulating, such as the sun salutation and the warrior pose, can help to balance Kapha and promote energy and motivation. Meditation is also effective for balancing Kapha, as it helps to promote emotional stability and endurance.

Ayurvedic Body Types

1. In Ayurveda, each individual is believed to have a unique combination of the three doshas: Vata, Pitta, and Kapha. This unique combination is known as the individual's Prakriti, or Ayurvedic body type. Understanding your Ayurvedic body type can help you make better lifestyle choices and maintain good health.

2. There are seven Ayurvedic body types: Vata, Pitta, Kapha, Vata-Pitta, Pitta-Kapha, Kapha-Vata, and Tridoshic. Each body type has its own unique characteristics and tendencies, and understanding your body type can help you understand your strengths and weaknesses.

Vata Body Type:

People with a Vata body type tend to be thin and have dry skin and hair. They are often creative, enthusiastic, and have a quick mind. When Vata is out of balance, however, people may experience anxiety, nervousness, insomnia, and digestive issues.

Pitta Body Type:

People with a Pitta body type tend to have a medium build, oily skin and hair, and a tendency to feel hot. They are often intelligent, ambitious, and confident. When Pitta is out of balance, however, people may experience anger, inflammation, and skin issues.

Kapha Body Type:

People with a Kapha body type tend to have a heavier build, soft skin and hair, and a tendency to feel cold. They are often calm, loving, and nurturing. When Kapha is out of balance, however, people may experience lethargy, weight gain, and respiratory issues.

Vata-Pitta Body Type:

People with a Vata-Pitta body type have a combination of the characteristics of both Vata and Pitta. They tend to have a thin build, dry skin and hair, and a tendency to feel hot. They are often creative, enthusiastic, intelligent, and ambitious.

Pitta-Kapha Body Type:

People with a Pitta-Kapha body type have a combination of the characteristics of both Pitta and Kapha. They tend to have a medium build, oily skin and hair, and a tendency to feel hot and cold at the same time. They are often intelligent, confident, loving, and nurturing.

Kapha-Vata Body Type:

People with a Kapha-Vata body type have a combination of the characteristics of both Kapha and Vata. They tend to have a heavier build, dry skin and hair, and a tendency to feel cold and anxious. They are often calm, loving, nurturing, and creative.

Tridoshic Body Type:

3. People with a Tridoshic body type have an equal balance of all three doshas: Vata, Pitta, and Kapha. They tend to have a balanced build, skin, and hair, and are often adaptable, flexible, and open-minded.

Knowing your Ayurvedic body type can help you make better lifestyle choices, such as choosing the right foods, exercise, and other daily habits that suit your unique needs. Ayurvedic treatments are tailored to each individual's body type, so understanding your Prakriti can help you find the right treatments for any health issues you may be experiencing.

Determining your dosha

1. Ayurveda recognizes that each person has a unique combination of the three doshas: Vata, Pitta, and Kapha. Determining your dosha can help you understand your body type and tailor your lifestyle choices accordingly.

There are several methods of determining your dosha, including a self-assessment, a consultation with an Ayurvedic practitioner, and pulse diagnosis.

Self-assessment is a simple and accessible way to determine your dosha. By answering a series of questions about your physical and emotional characteristics, tendencies, and preferences, you can get a general idea of your dosha. However, it is important to remember that self-assessment may not be entirely accurate, as it is subjective and can be influenced by personal biases.

Consulting with an Ayurvedic practitioner is a more thorough and accurate way to determine your dosha. An Ayurvedic practitioner can take into account not only your physical and emotional characteristics but also your medical history, family history, and lifestyle habits. A practitioner can also use specialized diagnostic tools, such as tongue and pulse diagnosis, to determine your dosha.

Pulse diagnosis is a unique diagnostic tool used in Ayurveda. By feeling the pulse in different locations on the wrist, an Ayurvedic practitioner can determine the balance of the three doshas in the body. The pulse is felt in three positions, corresponding to Vata, Pitta, and Kapha. The strength, rhythm, and qualities of the pulse in each position can indicate the balance of the corresponding dosha in the body.

Once you have determined your dosha, you can begin to make lifestyle choices that support your body type. Ayurvedic treatments are tailored to each individual's dosha, so understanding your dosha can help you find the right treatments for any health issues you may be experiencing.

For example, if you have a Pitta constitution, you may benefit from cooling foods and herbs, such as cucumber and coriander. You may also benefit from practices that promote relaxation and calmness, such as meditation and yoga.

If you have a Kapha constitution, you may benefit from invigorating foods and herbs, such as ginger and black pepper. You may also benefit from practices that promote movement and energy, such as cardio exercise and stimulating yoga poses.

If you have a Vata constitution, you may benefit from grounding foods and herbs, such as root vegetables and ashwagandha. You may also benefit from practices that promote stability and relaxation, such as restorative yoga and meditation.

In addition to diet and lifestyle changes, Ayurvedic treatments for imbalances in the doshas may include herbal remedies, massage, and other practices. Ayurvedic treatments are aimed at restoring balance to the doshas and promoting overall health and wellbeing.

Balancing your dosha

In Ayurveda, the three doshas - Vata, Pitta, and Kapha - are believed to be the fundamental principles that govern our bodies and minds. Each individual has a unique combination of these three doshas, known as their Prakriti. When the doshas are in balance, we experience good health and wellbeing. However, imbalances in the doshas can lead to various health issues. Here are some tips for balancing your dosha:

1. Eat a balanced diet: Ayurveda recommends eating a balanced diet that suits your dosha. For example, if you have a Pitta constitution, you may benefit from cooling foods such as cucumber, watermelon, and coconut. On the other hand, if you have a Kapha constitution, you may benefit from invigorating foods such as ginger, black pepper, and garlic. A balanced diet that includes fresh fruits and vegetables, whole grains, and lean proteins can help balance all three doshas.

2. Practice yoga: Yoga is an ancient practice that can help balance the doshas. Certain yoga poses are beneficial for each dosha. For example, if you have a Vata constitution, you may benefit from grounding poses such as Warrior II and Tree pose. If you have a Pitta constitution, you may benefit from cooling poses such as Camel pose and Forward Fold. And if you have a Kapha constitution, you may benefit from stimulating poses such as Sun Salutation and Locust pose.

3. Practice meditation: Meditation is a powerful tool for balancing the doshas. It can help reduce stress, calm the mind, and promote relaxation. Different meditation techniques may be more beneficial for each dosha. For example, if you have a Vata constitution, you may benefit from guided meditation or visualization techniques. If you have a Pitta constitution, you may benefit from chanting or mantra meditation. And if you have a Kapha constitution, you may benefit from breathwork or pranayama techniques.

4. Use herbal remedies: Ayurveda uses a variety of herbal remedies to balance the doshas. For example, if you have a Vata constitution, you may benefit from herbs such as ashwagandha and licorice root. If you have a Pitta constitution, you may benefit from herbs such as neem and brahmi. And if you have a Kapha constitution, you may benefit from herbs such as ginger and turmeric.

5. Practice self-care: Practicing self-care is essential for balancing the doshas. Self-care practices such as massage, aromatherapy, and taking relaxing baths can help reduce stress and promote relaxation. Each dosha may benefit from different self-care practices. For example, if you have a Vata constitution, you may benefit from self-massage with warm oil. If you have a Pitta constitution, you may benefit from aromatherapy with cooling essential oils such as peppermint and eucalyptus. And if you have a Kapha constitution, you may benefit from taking a warm bath with stimulating essential oils such as rosemary and juniper.

6. Get enough rest: Getting enough rest is crucial for balancing the doshas. Ayurveda recommends getting 7-8 hours of sleep each night. Each dosha may benefit from different sleep practices. For example, if you have a Vata constitution, you may benefit from going to bed and waking up at the same time each day to establish a routine. If you have a Pitta constitution, you may benefit from avoiding stimulating activities before bed and practicing relaxation techniques. And if you have a Kapha constitution, you may benefit from waking up early and practicing invigorating activities such as yoga and exercise.

Dosha-specific routines and lifestyle recommendations

Ayurveda recognizes that each individual has a unique combination of the three doshas - Vata, Pitta, and Kapha. Understanding your dosha can help you make lifestyle choices that support your unique constitution. Here are some dosha-specific routines and lifestyle recommendations:

Vata Dosha:

1. Stick to a routine: Vata dosha benefits from a consistent daily routine, with meals, exercise, and sleep at the same time each day.

2. Keep warm: Vata dosha tends to feel cold, so it is important to keep warm with warm clothing, blankets, and warm drinks.

3. Eat warm, nourishing foods: Vata dosha benefits from warm, nourishing foods such as soups, stews, and cooked grains. Avoid cold, raw foods.

4. Get enough rest: Vata dosha benefits from getting enough rest, as it can help calm the mind and reduce anxiety. Aim for 7-8 hours of sleep each night.

5. Practice gentle exercise: Vata dosha benefits from gentle exercise such as yoga, walking, and swimming.

6. Use grounding essential oils: Vata dosha benefits from using grounding essential oils such as lavender, sandalwood, and frankincense.

Pitta Dosha:

7. Stay cool: Pitta dosha benefits from staying cool, especially in hot weather. Wear light, breathable clothing and stay in the shade.

8. Eat cooling foods: Pitta dosha benefits from cooling foods such as cucumber, watermelon, and coconut. Avoid spicy and acidic foods.

9. Practice relaxation techniques: Pitta dosha benefits from practicing relaxation techniques such as meditation, deep breathing, and yoga.

10. Avoid excessive stimulation: Pitta dosha can be easily overstimulated, so it is important to avoid excessive screen time, loud noises, and bright lights.

11. Exercise in moderation: Pitta dosha benefits from moderate exercise such as walking, cycling, and yoga.

12. Use cooling essential oils: Pitta dosha benefits from using cooling essential oils such as peppermint, rose, and sandalwood.

Kapha Dosha:

13. Stay active: Kapha dosha benefits from regular exercise such as jogging, cycling, and dancing.

14. Eat stimulating foods: Kapha dosha benefits from stimulating foods such as ginger, garlic, and black pepper. Avoid heavy, oily foods.

15. Get enough rest: Kapha dosha benefits from getting enough rest, but too much sleep can exacerbate Kapha qualities. Aim for 7-8 hours of sleep each night.

16. Practice invigorating techniques: Kapha dosha benefits from invigorating techniques such as dry brushing, deep breathing, and yoga.

17. Avoid excess sweet and salty foods: Kapha dosha tends to have a sweet tooth and can easily overindulge in sweet and salty foods. Practice moderation in these foods.

18. Use stimulating essential oils: Kapha dosha benefits from using stimulating essential oils such as rosemary, eucalyptus, and bergamot.

Ayurvedic Nutrition and Diet

Ayurveda recognizes that diet plays a crucial role in promoting health and wellbeing. Ayurvedic nutrition and diet are based on the principles of balancing the three doshas - Vata, Pitta, and Kapha - and promoting optimal digestion and assimilation of nutrients. Here are some key principles of Ayurvedic nutrition and diet:

1. Eat according to your dosha: Ayurveda recognizes that each person has a unique combination of the three doshas, and therefore, each person's dietary needs are also unique. Eating according to your dosha can help balance the doshas and promote optimal health. For example, if you have a Pitta constitution, you may benefit from cooling foods such as cucumber, watermelon, and coconut. If you have a Vata constitution, you may benefit from grounding foods such as root vegetables and whole grains.

2. Eat fresh, whole foods: Ayurveda emphasizes the importance of eating fresh, whole foods that are minimally processed. Fresh, whole foods are easier to digest and contain more nutrients than processed foods. In Ayurveda, food is considered a form of medicine, and fresh, whole foods are seen as the most potent form of medicine.

3. Eat according to the seasons: Ayurveda recognizes that our dietary needs change with the seasons. Eating seasonally can help balance the doshas and promote optimal health. For example, in the summer, it is beneficial to eat cooling foods such as watermelon and cucumber, while in the winter, it is beneficial to eat warming foods such as soups and stews.

4. Favor certain tastes: Ayurveda recognizes six tastes - sweet, sour, salty, pungent, bitter, and astringent - and recommends favoring certain tastes depending on your dosha. For example, if you have a Pitta constitution, you may benefit from favoring sweet, bitter, and astringent tastes, while avoiding sour, salty, and pungent tastes.

5. Pay attention to digestion: Ayurveda recognizes the importance of optimal digestion for overall health and wellbeing. To promote optimal digestion, Ayurveda recommends eating in a calm, relaxed environment, chewing food thoroughly, and avoiding overeating. Eating a balanced diet that suits your dosha can also help promote optimal digestion.

6. Use spices and herbs: Ayurveda recognizes the medicinal properties of spices and herbs and recommends using them liberally in cooking. Spices and herbs can help balance the doshas, improve digestion, and enhance the flavor of foods. For example, ginger can help improve digestion and reduce inflammation, while turmeric can help balance the doshas and reduce inflammation.

7. Avoid processed foods: Ayurveda recommends avoiding processed foods, which are often high in preservatives, artificial flavors, and chemicals. Processed foods can be difficult to digest and can disrupt the balance of the doshas.

The six tastes and their effects on the doshas

Ayurveda recognizes six tastes - sweet, sour, salty, pungent, bitter, and astringent - and their effects on the doshas. Each taste has a specific effect on the doshas, and eating a balanced diet that includes all six tastes can help balance the doshas and promote optimal health. Here are the six tastes and their effects on the doshas:

1. Sweet taste: The sweet taste is nourishing and grounding and has a balancing effect on Vata and Pitta doshas. However, too much sweet taste can exacerbate Kapha dosha. Sweet foods include fruits, grains, and dairy products.

2. Sour taste: The sour taste is stimulating and has a balancing effect on Vata dosha. However, too much sour taste can exacerbate Pitta and Kapha doshas. Sour foods include citrus fruits, yogurt, and vinegar.

3. Salty taste: The salty taste is hydrating and has a balancing effect on Vata dosha. However, too much salty taste can exacerbate Pitta and Kapha doshas. Salty foods include salt, seaweed, and cured meats.

4. Pungent taste: The pungent taste is heating and has a balancing effect on Kapha dosha. However, too much pungent taste can exacerbate Pitta and Vata doshas. Pungent foods include chili peppers, ginger, and garlic.

5. Bitter taste: The bitter taste is detoxifying and has a balancing effect on Pitta and Kapha doshas. However, too much bitter taste can exacerbate Vata dosha. Bitter foods include leafy greens, turmeric, and bitter melon.

6. Astringent taste: The astringent taste is drying and has a balancing effect on Kapha dosha. However, too much astringent taste can exacerbate Vata and Pitta doshas. Astringent foods include legumes, pomegranate, and cranberries.

In Ayurveda, it is recommended to eat a balanced diet that includes all six tastes. Eating a variety of foods that include different tastes can help balance the doshas and promote optimal health. For example, a meal that includes rice (sweet taste), lemon (sour taste), salted nuts (salty taste), ginger (pungent taste), spinach (bitter taste), and beans (astringent taste) can help balance the doshas and promote optimal digestion and assimilation of nutrients.

In addition to including all six tastes in your diet, Ayurveda recommends favoring certain tastes depending on your dosha. Here are some guidelines for each dosha:

7. Vata dosha: Favor sweet, sour, and salty tastes and avoid bitter, pungent, and astringent tastes.

8. Pitta dosha: Favor sweet, bitter, and astringent tastes and avoid sour, salty, and pungent tastes.

9. Kapha dosha: Favor pungent, bitter, and astringent tastes and avoid sweet, sour, and salty tastes.

Ayurvedic food guidelines for optimal health

Ayurveda recognizes that food plays a crucial role in promoting optimal health and wellbeing. Ayurvedic food guidelines are based on the principles of balancing the doshas and promoting optimal digestion and assimilation of nutrients. Here are some key Ayurvedic food guidelines for optimal health:

1. Eat according to your dosha: Ayurveda recognizes that each person has a unique combination of the three doshas - Vata, Pitta, and Kapha - and therefore, each person's dietary needs are also unique. Eating according to your dosha can help balance the doshas and promote optimal health. For example, if you have a Pitta constitution, you may benefit from cooling foods such as cucumber, watermelon, and coconut. If you have a Vata constitution, you may benefit from grounding foods such as root vegetables and whole grains.

2. Eat fresh, whole foods: Ayurveda emphasizes the importance of eating fresh, whole foods that are minimally processed. Fresh, whole foods are easier to digest and contain more nutrients than processed foods. In Ayurveda, food is considered a form of medicine, and fresh, whole foods are seen as the most potent form of medicine.

3. Eat warm, cooked foods: Ayurveda recognizes that raw foods can be difficult to digest, especially for those with a weak digestive system. Eating warm, cooked foods can help improve digestion and assimilation of nutrients. Cooked foods are also easier on the digestive system than raw foods.

4. Eat in a calm, relaxed environment: Ayurveda recognizes the importance of eating in a calm, relaxed environment. Eating in a calm, relaxed environment can help promote optimal digestion and assimilation of nutrients. Avoid eating in a hurry, in front of the TV, or while stressed.

5. Favor certain tastes: Ayurveda recognizes six tastes - sweet, sour, salty, pungent, bitter, and astringent - and recommends favoring certain tastes depending on your dosha. For example, if you have a Pitta constitution, you may benefit from favoring sweet, bitter, and astringent tastes, while avoiding sour, salty, and pungent tastes.

6. Use spices and herbs: Ayurveda recognizes the medicinal properties of spices and herbs and recommends using them liberally in cooking. Spices and herbs can help balance the doshas, improve digestion, and enhance the flavor of foods. For example, ginger can help improve digestion and reduce inflammation, while turmeric can help balance the doshas and reduce inflammation.

7. Avoid processed foods: Ayurveda recommends avoiding processed foods, which are often high in preservatives, artificial flavors, and chemicals. Processed foods can be difficult to digest and can disrupt the balance of the doshas.

8. Eat according to the seasons: Ayurveda recognizes that our dietary needs change with the seasons. Eating seasonally can help balance the doshas and promote optimal health. For example, in the summer, it is beneficial to eat cooling foods such as watermelon and cucumber, while in the winter, it is beneficial to eat warming foods such as soups and stews.

9. Eat mindfully: Ayurveda recognizes the importance of eating mindfully. Eating mindfully can help promote optimal digestion and assimilation of nutrients. Take the time to savor each bite, chew food thoroughly, and avoid overeating.

Meal planning and preparation for your dosha

Meal planning and preparation are essential aspects of an Ayurvedic lifestyle. Ayurveda recognizes that each person has a unique combination of the three doshas - Vata, Pitta, and Kapha - and therefore, each person's dietary needs are also unique. Meal planning and preparation for your dosha can help balance the doshas and promote optimal health. Here are some key tips for meal planning and preparation for your dosha:

1. Determine your dosha: Before you start meal planning and preparation, it is essential to determine your dosha. You can take an online dosha quiz or consult with an Ayurvedic practitioner to determine your dosha. Once you know your dosha, you can plan and prepare meals that are tailored to your unique needs.

2. Create a meal plan: Creating a meal plan can help you stay organized and ensure that you are eating a balanced diet. Start by planning out your meals for the week, including breakfast, lunch, dinner, and snacks. Consider incorporating all six tastes - sweet, sour, salty, pungent, bitter, and astringent - into your meals to help balance the doshas.

3. Shop for fresh, whole foods: Once you have your meal plan, make a shopping list of the ingredients you need. Look for fresh, whole foods that are minimally processed. Fresh, whole foods are easier to digest and contain more nutrients than processed foods.

4. Use spices and herbs: Spices and herbs are an essential part of Ayurvedic cooking. They can help balance the doshas, improve digestion, and enhance the flavor of foods. Consider stocking your pantry with a variety of spices and herbs, such as ginger, turmeric, cumin, coriander, and fennel.

5. Cook with your dosha in mind: When preparing meals, consider your dosha and choose ingredients and cooking methods that balance your dosha. For example, if you have a Vata constitution, you may benefit from warming, grounding foods such as root vegetables and whole grains. If you have a Pitta constitution, you may benefit from cooling, hydrating foods such as cucumber and watermelon.

6. Cook with love and intention: Ayurveda recognizes that the energy we put into our food affects its quality and our digestion. When preparing meals, cook with love and intention, and avoid cooking when you are stressed or upset.

7. Eat in a calm, relaxed environment: Eating in a calm, relaxed environment is essential for optimal digestion and assimilation of nutrients. Create a peaceful, inviting space to enjoy your meals and avoid eating in a hurry, in front of the TV, or while stressed.

8. Practice mindful eating: Mindful eating can help promote optimal digestion and assimilation of nutrients. Take the time to savor each bite, chew food thoroughly, and avoid overeating.

9. Experiment with new recipes: Experimenting with new recipes can help keep your meals interesting and enjoyable. Look for Ayurvedic cookbooks or online resources for inspiration and try new ingredients and cooking methods.

Ayurvedic Herbs and Supplements

Ayurveda recognizes the medicinal properties of herbs and supplements and uses them to promote optimal health and wellbeing. Ayurvedic herbs and supplements can help balance the doshas, improve digestion, boost immunity, and support overall health. Here are some key Ayurvedic herbs and supplements:

1. Ashwagandha: Ashwagandha is an adaptogenic herb that helps the body adapt to stress. It is also known for its ability to balance the doshas, support the immune system, and promote overall vitality.

2. Turmeric: Turmeric is a powerful anti-inflammatory herb that is commonly used in Ayurvedic medicine. It is known for its ability to balance the doshas, support digestion, and promote healthy skin.

3. Triphala: Triphala is a blend of three fruits - amla, haritaki, and bibhitaki - that is commonly used in Ayurvedic medicine to support digestion, improve immunity, and promote overall health.

4. Brahmi: Brahmi is an herb that is commonly used in Ayurvedic medicine to support cognitive function, reduce stress, and promote overall wellbeing.

5. Tulsi: Tulsi, also known as holy basil, is an herb that is commonly used in Ayurvedic medicine to reduce stress, boost immunity, and support overall health.

6. Ginger: Ginger is a digestive herb that is commonly used in Ayurvedic medicine to support digestion, reduce inflammation, and boost immunity.

7. Guggulu: Guggulu is a resin that is commonly used in Ayurvedic medicine to support healthy cholesterol levels, reduce inflammation, and promote overall health.

8. Shatavari: Shatavari is an adaptogenic herb that is commonly used in Ayurvedic medicine to support women's health, balance the hormones, and promote overall vitality.

9. Neem: Neem is an herb that is commonly used in Ayurvedic medicine to support healthy skin, boost immunity, and promote overall health.

In addition to these Ayurvedic herbs, there are also Ayurvedic supplements that can help support optimal health. Here are some key Ayurvedic supplements:

10. Triphala: Triphala is a supplement that contains the same blend of three fruits - amla, haritaki, and bibhitaki - as the Ayurvedic herb triphala. Triphala supplements are commonly used in Ayurvedic medicine to support digestion, improve immunity, and promote overall health.

11. Digestive enzymes: Digestive enzymes are supplements that help support digestion and assimilation of nutrients. They are commonly used in Ayurvedic medicine to support optimal digestion and reduce digestive issues such as bloating and gas.

12. Probiotics: Probiotics are supplements that contain beneficial bacteria that help support gut health and immunity. They are commonly used in Ayurvedic medicine to support optimal digestion and overall health.

13. Omega-3 fatty acids: Omega-3 fatty acids are supplements that are commonly used in Ayurvedic medicine to support heart health, brain health, and overall health.

14. Vitamin D: Vitamin D is a supplement that is commonly used in Ayurvedic medicine to support bone health, immune function, and overall health.

The role of herbs in Ayurveda

Herbs play a significant role in Ayurveda, an ancient system of medicine that originated in India over 5,000 years ago. Ayurveda recognizes the medicinal properties of herbs and uses them to promote optimal health and wellbeing. Here are some key aspects of the role of herbs in Ayurveda:

1. Balancing the doshas: Ayurveda recognizes that each person has a unique combination of the three doshas - Vata, Pitta, and Kapha - and imbalances in the doshas can lead to illness and disease. Herbs are used in Ayurveda to balance the doshas and restore health. For example, warming herbs like ginger and cinnamon can balance Vata, cooling herbs like coriander and fennel can balance Pitta, and grounding herbs like ashwagandha and licorice can balance Kapha.

2. Improving digestion: Ayurveda recognizes that proper digestion is essential for optimal health and wellbeing. Herbs are used in Ayurveda to support digestion and promote the assimilation of nutrients. For example, digestive herbs like ginger, cardamom, and cumin can help improve digestion, reduce bloating and gas, and soothe the digestive tract.

3. Boosting immunity: Ayurveda recognizes that a strong immune system is essential for optimal health and wellbeing. Herbs are used in Ayurveda to boost immunity and promote overall health. For example, immune-boosting herbs like turmeric, tulsi, and neem can help support the immune system, reduce inflammation, and promote overall health.

4. Supporting detoxification: Ayurveda recognizes that toxins can accumulate in the body and lead to illness and disease. Herbs are used in Ayurveda to support detoxification and promote the elimination of toxins from the body. For example, detoxifying herbs like triphala and dandelion can help support liver function, promote healthy bowel movements, and eliminate toxins from the body.

5. Promoting mental and emotional balance: Ayurveda recognizes that mental and emotional balance is essential for optimal health and wellbeing. Herbs are used in Ayurveda to promote mental and emotional balance and support the nervous system. For example, calming herbs like brahmi and ashwagandha can help reduce stress, promote relaxation, and support mental and emotional balance.

6. Enhancing overall vitality: Ayurveda recognizes that overall vitality is essential for optimal health and wellbeing. Herbs are used in Ayurveda to enhance overall vitality and promote longevity. For example, adaptogenic herbs like ashwagandha and shatavari can help the body adapt to stress, support the immune system, and enhance overall vitality.

Common Ayurvedic herbs and their benefits

Ayurveda is an ancient system of medicine that recognizes the medicinal properties of herbs and uses them to promote optimal health and wellbeing. Ayurvedic herbs are known for their therapeutic properties and have been used for centuries to support digestion, boost immunity, promote mental and emotional balance, and enhance overall vitality. Here are some of the most common Ayurvedic herbs and their benefits:

1. Ashwagandha: Ashwagandha is an adaptogenic herb that helps the body adapt to stress. It is known for its ability to balance the doshas, support the immune system, and promote overall vitality. Ashwagandha has also been shown to improve cognitive function, reduce inflammation, and promote healthy sleep.

2. Turmeric: Turmeric is a powerful anti-inflammatory herb that is commonly used in Ayurvedic medicine. It is known for its ability to balance the doshas, support digestion, and promote healthy skin. Turmeric has also been shown to support brain function, reduce the risk of heart disease, and promote overall health.

3. Triphala: Triphala is a blend of three fruits - amla, haritaki, and bibhitaki - that is commonly used in Ayurvedic medicine to support digestion, improve immunity, and promote overall health. Triphala is also known for its ability to promote healthy bowel movements, support liver function, and reduce inflammation.

4. Brahmi: Brahmi is an herb that is commonly used in Ayurvedic medicine to support cognitive function, reduce stress, and promote overall wellbeing. Brahmi has been shown to improve memory, reduce anxiety, and promote relaxation.

5. Tulsi: Tulsi, also known as holy basil, is an herb that is commonly used in Ayurvedic medicine to reduce stress, boost immunity, and support overall health. Tulsi has also been shown to reduce inflammation, improve digestion, and promote healthy skin.

6. Ginger: Ginger is a digestive herb that is commonly used in Ayurvedic medicine to support digestion, reduce inflammation, and boost immunity. Ginger has also been shown to improve brain function, reduce muscle pain, and promote healthy aging.

7. Guggulu: Guggulu is a resin that is commonly used in Ayurvedic medicine to support healthy cholesterol levels, reduce inflammation, and promote overall health. Guggulu has also been shown to support healthy weight management, reduce acne, and improve joint health.

8. Shatavari: Shatavari is an adaptogenic herb that is commonly used in Ayurvedic medicine to support women's health, balance the hormones, and promote overall vitality. Shatavari has been shown to improve fertility, reduce symptoms of menopause, and support lactation in nursing mothers.

9. Neem: Neem is an herb that is commonly used in Ayurvedic medicine to support healthy skin, boost immunity, and promote overall health. Neem has also been shown to reduce inflammation, support healthy blood sugar levels, and promote healthy digestion.

Guidelines for choosing and using Ayurvedic supplements

Ayurveda, an ancient system of medicine, recognizes the medicinal properties of herbs and uses them to promote optimal health and wellbeing. Ayurvedic supplements are a popular way to incorporate herbs into our daily routine and support our health and wellbeing. Here are some guidelines for choosing and using Ayurvedic supplements:

1. Consult with an Ayurvedic practitioner: Before choosing and using Ayurvedic supplements, it is important to consult with a qualified Ayurvedic practitioner. They can help you identify your dosha, recommend supplements that are appropriate for your constitution, and provide guidance on safe and effective use.

2. Choose high-quality supplements: When choosing Ayurvedic supplements, it is important to choose high-quality products that are free from contaminants and meet the standards of good manufacturing practices. Look for supplements that are certified organic, non-GMO, and free from artificial additives.

3. Start with a low dose: When starting a new supplement, it is important to start with a low dose and gradually increase it over time. This can help your body adjust to the supplement and minimize the risk of side effects.

4. Take supplements with food: Many Ayurvedic supplements are best taken with food to enhance absorption and minimize the risk of digestive upset. Check the label of the supplement for specific instructions on how to take it.

5. Be consistent: To experience the full benefits of Ayurvedic supplements, it is important to take them consistently over time. Set a schedule for taking your supplements and stick to it.

6. Monitor for side effects: While Ayurvedic supplements are generally safe, it is important to monitor for any potential side effects. If you experience any adverse effects, stop taking the supplement and consult with your Ayurvedic practitioner.

7. Avoid interactions with medications: Some Ayurvedic supplements may interact with medications or other supplements. It is important to consult with your healthcare provider before adding any new supplements to your regimen to avoid potential interactions.

8. Consider the source of the supplement: When choosing Ayurvedic supplements, consider the source of the supplement. Look for supplements that are sustainably sourced and support fair trade practices.

Ayurvedic Detoxification and Cleansing

Ayurveda, an ancient system of medicine, recognizes the importance of detoxification and cleansing to support optimal health and wellbeing. Ayurvedic detoxification and cleansing practices are designed to remove toxins from the body, promote digestion, boost immunity, and enhance overall vitality. Here are some of the most common Ayurvedic detoxification and cleansing practices:

1. Abhyanga: Abhyanga is an Ayurvedic practice that involves massaging warm oil onto the skin. This practice is believed to help remove toxins from the body, improve circulation, and promote relaxation. To practice abhyanga, warm up some sesame or coconut oil and massage it onto your skin in circular motions.

2. Neti: Neti is an Ayurvedic practice that involves using a neti pot to flush out the nasal passages with saline water. This practice is believed to help remove excess mucus, relieve sinus congestion, and promote respiratory health. To practice neti, fill a neti pot with warm saline water, tilt your head to one side, and pour the water into one nostril. The water will flow out of the other nostril, carrying any excess mucus with it.

3. Tongue scraping: Tongue scraping is an Ayurvedic practice that involves using a tongue scraper to remove toxins and bacteria from the tongue. This practice is believed to help improve digestion, freshen breath, and promote overall oral health. To practice tongue scraping, use a tongue scraper to gently scrape the surface of your tongue from back to front.

4. Triphala: Triphala is an Ayurvedic herbal formula that is commonly used to support digestive health and promote detoxification. Triphala is a blend of three fruits - amla, haritaki, and bibhitaki - that is believed to help remove toxins from the body, support healthy bowel movements, and promote overall health.

5. Fasting: Fasting is an Ayurvedic practice that involves abstaining from food for a period of time. This practice is believed to help give the digestive system a break, promote detoxification, and enhance overall vitality. To practice fasting, choose a day or two each week to eat only light meals or abstain from food altogether.

6. Ayurvedic teas: Ayurvedic teas are blends of herbs that are designed to promote digestion, boost immunity, and support detoxification. Some common Ayurvedic teas include ginger tea, tulsi tea, and licorice tea. These teas can be enjoyed throughout the day to support overall health and wellbeing.

7. Panchakarma: Panchakarma is an Ayurvedic cleansing and detoxification program that involves a series of therapies and treatments. This program is designed to remove deep-seated toxins from the body, promote digestive health, and enhance overall vitality. Panchakarma typically involves a combination of massage, herbal remedies, and dietary changes.

The importance of detoxification in Ayurveda

Ayurveda, an ancient system of medicine, recognizes the importance of detoxification to support optimal health and wellbeing. Detoxification is the process of removing toxins from the body, which can accumulate due to poor diet, lifestyle choices, environmental pollutants, and other factors. In Ayurveda, detoxification is considered a cornerstone of health and is believed to promote digestion, boost immunity, and enhance overall vitality. Here are some of the reasons why detoxification is so important in Ayurveda:

1. Removes toxins from the body: Detoxification is important because it helps remove toxins from the body. Toxins can accumulate in the body over time due to poor diet, lifestyle choices, environmental pollutants, and other factors. These toxins can interfere with the normal functioning of the body and contribute to a range of health problems. By removing these toxins, detoxification can help restore balance to the body and promote optimal health and wellbeing.

2. Supports digestion: Detoxification is important for digestion because it helps remove ama, a toxic substance that can accumulate in the digestive tract. Ama is believed to be the root cause of many digestive problems, including constipation, bloating, and gas. By removing ama from the digestive tract, detoxification can help improve digestion and promote overall digestive health.

3. Boosts immunity: Detoxification is important for immunity because it helps remove toxins that can compromise the immune system. When the body is exposed to toxins, the immune system can become overtaxed and weakened, making it more susceptible to infections and other health problems. By removing toxins from the body, detoxification can help strengthen the immune system and enhance overall immunity.

4. Enhances overall vitality: Detoxification is important for overall vitality because it helps remove toxins that can interfere with the normal functioning of the body. When the body is burdened with toxins, it can become sluggish, tired, and prone to illness. By removing toxins from the body, detoxification can help restore energy and vitality, promoting optimal health and wellbeing.

5. Balances the doshas: Detoxification is important for balancing the doshas, the three principles of Ayurveda that govern the functioning of the body. When the doshas are out of balance, the body can become prone to a range of health problems. By removing toxins from the body, detoxification can help balance the doshas, promoting overall health and wellbeing.

In Ayurveda, there are several ways to support detoxification, including diet, lifestyle choices, and specific Ayurvedic therapies. Some common Ayurvedic detoxification practices include fasting, tongue scraping, abhyanga (oil massage), and panchakarma, a comprehensive Ayurvedic detoxification program. By incorporating these practices into our daily routine, we can support optimal health and wellbeing by promoting detoxification, boosting digestion, enhancing immunity, restoring energy and vitality, and balancing the doshas.

Ayurvedic cleansing techniques

Ayurveda, an ancient system of medicine, recognizes the importance of cleansing techniques to support optimal health and wellbeing. Cleansing techniques are designed to remove toxins and waste from the body, promoting digestion, enhancing energy and vitality, and supporting overall health. In Ayurveda, there are several cleansing techniques that are used to promote optimal health and wellbeing. Here are some of the most common Ayurvedic cleansing techniques:

1. Abhyanga: Abhyanga is an Ayurvedic practice that involves massaging warm oil onto the skin. This practice is believed to help remove toxins from the body, improve circulation, and promote relaxation. To practice abhyanga, warm up some sesame or coconut oil and massage it onto your skin in circular motions.

2. Neti: Neti is an Ayurvedic practice that involves using a neti pot to flush out the nasal passages with saline water. This practice is believed to help remove excess mucus, relieve sinus congestion, and promote respiratory health. To practice neti, fill a neti pot with warm saline water, tilt your head to one side, and pour the water into one nostril. The water will flow out of the other nostril, carrying any excess mucus with it.

3. Tongue scraping: Tongue scraping is an Ayurvedic practice that involves using a tongue scraper to remove toxins and bacteria from the tongue. This practice is believed to help improve digestion, freshen breath, and promote overall oral health. To practice tongue scraping, use a tongue scraper to gently scrape the surface of your tongue from back to front.

4. Triphala: Triphala is an Ayurvedic herbal formula that is commonly used to support digestive health and promote detoxification. Triphala is a blend of three fruits - amla, haritaki, and bibhitaki - that is believed to help remove toxins from the body, support healthy bowel movements, and promote overall health.

5. Fasting: Fasting is an Ayurvedic practice that involves abstaining from food for a period of time. This practice is believed to help give the digestive system a break, promote detoxification, and enhance overall vitality. To practice fasting, choose a day or two each week to eat only light meals or abstain from food altogether.

6. Ayurvedic teas: Ayurvedic teas are blends of herbs that are designed to promote digestion, boost immunity, and support detoxification. Some common Ayurvedic teas include ginger tea, tulsi tea, and licorice tea. These teas can be enjoyed throughout the day to support overall health and wellbeing.

7. Panchakarma: Panchakarma is an Ayurvedic cleansing and detoxification program that involves a series of therapies and treatments. This program is designed to remove deep-seated toxins from the body, promote digestive health, and enhance overall vitality. Panchakarma typically involves a combination of massage, herbal remedies, and dietary changes.

Seasonal detoxification and rejuvenation

Ayurveda, an ancient system of medicine, recognizes the importance of seasonal detoxification and rejuvenation to support optimal health and wellbeing. In Ayurveda, each season is associated with different doshas and elements, and seasonal changes can have a profound effect on our health and wellbeing. Seasonal detoxification and rejuvenation practices are designed to help us adapt to these changes and promote optimal health and wellbeing. Here are some of the most common Ayurvedic practices for seasonal detoxification and rejuvenation:

1. Adjusting diet and lifestyle: One of the most important ways to support seasonal detoxification and rejuvenation is to adjust your diet and lifestyle to match the season. In Ayurveda, each season is associated with different foods, activities, and habits. For example, in the spring, it is recommended to eat lighter, more cleansing foods, such as leafy greens and bitter vegetables, and to engage in activities that promote cleansing and rejuvenation, such as yoga and meditation.

2. Seasonal cleansing practices: In addition to adjusting your diet and lifestyle, seasonal cleansing practices can also be helpful for promoting detoxification and rejuvenation. Some common seasonal cleansing practices include fasting, herbal remedies, and body treatments, such as massage and steam baths. These practices are designed to help remove toxins from the body, boost digestion, and promote overall health and wellbeing.

3. Herbal remedies: In Ayurveda, herbal remedies are commonly used to support seasonal detoxification and rejuvenation. Herbs such as triphala, ashwagandha, and turmeric are believed to help remove toxins from the body, boost immunity, and promote overall health and wellbeing. These herbs can be taken in the form of teas, capsules, or powders.

4. Ayurvedic massage: Ayurvedic massage, also known as abhyanga, is a practice that involves massaging warm oil onto the skin. This practice is believed to help promote detoxification, boost circulation, and enhance overall health and wellbeing. During seasonal changes, it is especially important to incorporate Ayurvedic massage into your routine to support detoxification and rejuvenation.

5. Yoga and meditation: Yoga and meditation are practices that are commonly used in Ayurveda to promote overall health and wellbeing. These practices are believed to help reduce stress, boost immunity, and promote overall vitality. During seasonal changes, it is important to incorporate yoga and meditation into your routine to support detoxification and rejuvenation.

Ayurvedic Daily Routines (Dinacharya)

Ayurveda, an ancient system of medicine, recognizes the importance of daily routines, or dinacharya, to support optimal health and wellbeing. In Ayurveda, daily routines are designed to help us align with the natural rhythms of the day and promote optimal digestion, energy, and vitality. Here are some of the most common Ayurvedic daily routines:

1. Wake up early: Ayurveda recommends waking up early, ideally before sunrise, to align with the natural rhythms of the day. Waking up early helps promote energy and vitality, and allows us to take advantage of the peacefulness of the early morning hours.

2. Scrape the tongue: Tongue scraping is an Ayurvedic practice that involves using a tongue scraper to remove toxins and bacteria from the tongue. This practice is believed to help improve digestion, freshen breath, and promote overall oral health.

3. Brush teeth and rinse mouth: Brushing your teeth and rinsing your mouth is an important part of maintaining oral health and hygiene. In Ayurveda, it is recommended to use herbal toothpaste and mouthwash to support overall oral health.

4. Drink warm water: Drinking warm water first thing in the morning is believed to help stimulate digestion, promote detoxification, and enhance overall energy and vitality.

5. Practice yoga or exercise: Yoga and exercise are important practices in Ayurveda to promote overall health and wellbeing. These practices are believed to help reduce stress, boost immunity, and promote overall vitality.

6. Take a shower: Taking a shower is an important part of maintaining personal hygiene and promoting overall health and wellbeing. In Ayurveda, it is recommended to use warm water and natural, herbal soap to support optimal health and wellbeing.

7. Practice meditation: Meditation is an important practice in Ayurveda to promote relaxation, reduce stress, and enhance overall wellbeing. Practicing meditation daily can help promote mental clarity and emotional balance.

8. Eat a healthy breakfast: Eating a healthy breakfast is an important part of promoting optimal digestion and energy throughout the day. In Ayurveda, it is recommended to eat a breakfast that is easy to digest, such as warm oatmeal or a fruit smoothie.

9. Follow a regular meal schedule: Following a regular meal schedule is important in Ayurveda to promote optimal digestion and energy throughout the day. Eating meals at regular intervals helps support a healthy metabolism and promotes overall health and wellbeing.

10. Practice relaxation techniques before bed: Practicing relaxation techniques, such as reading or taking a warm bath, before bed can help promote restful sleep and enhance overall wellbeing.

The importance of daily routines in Ayurveda

Ayurveda, an ancient system of medicine, recognizes the importance of daily routines in promoting optimal health and wellbeing. In Ayurveda, daily routines, also known as dinacharya, are considered essential for maintaining balance and harmony within the body, mind, and spirit. These routines are designed to help us align with the natural rhythms of the day and promote optimal digestion, energy, and vitality.

One of the key principles of Ayurveda is that health is not just the absence of disease, but a state of complete physical, mental, and spiritual wellbeing. Daily routines in Ayurveda are designed to support this holistic approach to health, by promoting balance and harmony in all aspects of our being. Here are some of the key benefits of daily routines in Ayurveda:

1. Promotes optimal digestion: In Ayurveda, digestion is considered one of the most important factors in overall health and wellbeing. Daily routines, such as eating meals at regular intervals and practicing relaxation techniques before bed, help promote optimal digestion and prevent digestive problems.

2. Enhances energy and vitality: Daily routines in Ayurveda are designed to help us align with the natural rhythms of the day, promoting optimal energy and vitality. Waking up early, practicing yoga or exercise, and eating a healthy breakfast are just a few examples of Ayurvedic practices that can help enhance energy and vitality.

3. Reduces stress: Stress is a major contributor to many health problems, including digestive problems, insomnia, and anxiety. Daily routines, such as practicing meditation and relaxation techniques, can help reduce stress and promote overall mental and emotional wellbeing.

4. Boosts immunity: In Ayurveda, optimal health is dependent on a strong immune system. Daily routines, such as eating a healthy diet, getting regular exercise, and practicing relaxation techniques, can help boost immunity and prevent illness.

5. Supports emotional balance: Ayurveda recognizes the important connection between emotional and physical health. Daily routines, such as practicing meditation and relaxation techniques, can help promote emotional balance and prevent mood disorders.

In Ayurveda, there are many daily routines that are considered essential for promoting optimal health and wellbeing. Some of the most common Ayurvedic daily routines include:

6. Waking up early: Ayurveda recommends waking up early, ideally before sunrise, to align with the natural rhythms of the day and promote energy and vitality.

7. Tongue scraping: Tongue scraping is an Ayurvedic practice that involves using a tongue scraper to remove toxins and bacteria from the tongue. This practice is believed to help improve digestion, freshen breath, and promote overall oral health.

8. Drinking warm water: Drinking warm water first thing in the morning is believed to help stimulate digestion, promote detoxification, and enhance overall energy and vitality.

9. Practicing yoga or exercise: Yoga and exercise are important practices in Ayurveda to promote overall health and wellbeing. These practices are believed to help reduce stress, boost immunity, and promote overall vitality.

10. Eating a healthy breakfast: Eating a healthy breakfast is an important part of promoting optimal digestion and energy throughout the day. In Ayurveda, it is recommended to eat a breakfast that is easy to digest, such as warm oatmeal or a fruit smoothie.

11. Following a regular meal schedule: Following a regular meal schedule is important in Ayurveda to promote optimal digestion and energy throughout the day. Eating meals at regular intervals helps support a healthy metabolism and promotes overall health and wellbeing.

12. Practicing relaxation techniques before bed: Practicing relaxation techniques, such as reading or taking a warm bath, before bed can help promote restful sleep and enhance overall wellbeing.

Ayurvedic morning and evening routines

Ayurveda, the ancient system of medicine, emphasizes the importance of morning and evening routines to promote optimal health and wellbeing. In Ayurveda, these routines are known as dinacharya, and they are considered essential for maintaining balance and harmony within the body, mind, and spirit.

Morning Routine:

In Ayurveda, the morning routine is designed to help us align with the natural rhythms of the day and promote optimal energy and vitality. Here are some of the key practices that are typically included in an Ayurvedic morning routine:

1. Wake up early: Ayurveda recommends waking up early, ideally before sunrise, to align with the natural rhythms of the day and promote energy and vitality.

2. Tongue scraping: Tongue scraping is an Ayurvedic practice that involves using a tongue scraper to remove toxins and bacteria from the tongue. This practice is believed to help improve digestion, freshen breath, and promote overall oral health.

3. Drinking warm water: Drinking warm water first thing in the morning is believed to help stimulate digestion, promote detoxification, and enhance overall energy and vitality.

4. Practicing yoga or exercise: Yoga and exercise are important practices in Ayurveda to promote overall health and wellbeing. These practices are believed to help reduce stress, boost immunity, and promote overall vitality.

5. Meditation or Pranayama: Ayurveda recommends practicing meditation or pranayama in the morning to promote calmness and clarity of mind.

6. Abhyanga: Abhyanga is an Ayurvedic self-massage technique that involves using warm oil to massage the body. This practice is believed to promote relaxation, improve circulation, and enhance overall wellbeing.

7. Eating a healthy breakfast: Eating a healthy breakfast is an important part of promoting optimal digestion and energy throughout the day. In Ayurveda, it is recommended to eat a breakfast that is easy to digest, such as warm oatmeal or a fruit smoothie.

Evening Routine:

In Ayurveda, the evening routine is designed to help us wind down from the day and prepare for restful sleep. Here are some of the key practices that are typically included in an Ayurvedic evening routine:

8. Eating a light dinner: In Ayurveda, it is recommended to eat a light dinner that is easy to digest to promote restful sleep.

9. Practicing relaxation techniques: Practicing relaxation techniques, such as reading or taking a warm bath, before bed can help promote restful sleep and enhance overall wellbeing.

10. Unwinding and disconnecting: Ayurveda recommends disconnecting from technology and work-related activities at least one hour before bed to promote relaxation and reduce stress.

11. Abhyanga: Abhyanga is also recommended as an evening practice to promote relaxation and improve sleep.

12. Meditation or Pranayama: Practicing meditation or pranayama in the evening can help promote relaxation and prepare the mind and body for restful sleep.

13. Going to bed early: Ayurveda recommends going to bed early, ideally by 10 pm, to align with the natural rhythms of the day and promote restful sleep.

Benefits of Ayurvedic Morning and Evening Routines:

14. Promotes optimal digestion: Ayurvedic morning and evening routines are designed to promote optimal digestion and prevent digestive problems.

15. Enhances energy and vitality: Ayurvedic morning routines can help enhance energy and vitality for the day, while evening routines can help promote restful sleep and improve overall energy levels.

16. Reduces stress: Practicing relaxation techniques and disconnecting from technology in the evening can help reduce stress and promote relaxation.

17. Boosts immunity: Ayurvedic morning routines that include yoga or exercise can help boost immunity and prevent illness.

Promotes emotional balance:

Tailoring your daily routine to your dosha

In Ayurveda, tailoring your daily routine to your dosha is an important way to promote optimal health and wellbeing. Each dosha has unique characteristics and tendencies, and by understanding your own dosha, you can make choices in your daily routine that support your individual needs.

Vata Dosha:

If you have a predominant Vata dosha, you may be naturally creative, energetic, and adaptable, but may also be prone to anxiety, worry, and nervousness. To balance Vata dosha, it is important to create a sense of routine and stability in your daily life. Here are some recommendations for tailoring your daily routine to Vata dosha:

Wake up at the same time each day, ideally before sunrise.

Drink warm water with lemon in the morning to help promote digestion.

Eat warm, nourishing meals throughout the day, and avoid cold or raw foods.

Practice yoga or other gentle exercise to help ground and balance your energy.

Incorporate relaxation techniques such as meditation, deep breathing, or a warm bath into your evening routine.

Use warm, grounding essential oils such as sandalwood, ginger, or cedarwood.

Get regular massage or bodywork to help promote relaxation and reduce stress.

Pitta Dosha:

If you have a predominant Pitta dosha, you may be naturally confident, organized, and focused, but may also be prone to irritability, anger, and inflammation. To balance Pitta dosha, it is important to create a sense of calm and coolness in your daily life. Here are some recommendations for tailoring your daily routine to Pitta dosha:

Wake up early, ideally before sunrise.

Drink room temperature water with lime in the morning to help cool and hydrate your system.

Eat cooling, refreshing foods such as cucumber, watermelon, or mint.

Practice calming yoga or other forms of exercise such as swimming or walking.

Incorporate relaxation techniques such as meditation, visualization, or aromatherapy into your evening routine.

Use cooling essential oils such as peppermint, lavender, or rose.

Avoid overworking or overstimulating yourself, and allow time for rest and relaxation.

Kapha Dosha:

If you have a predominant Kapha dosha, you may be naturally calm, grounded, and nurturing, but may also be prone to lethargy, weight gain, and stagnation. To balance Kapha dosha, it is important to create a sense of movement and stimulation in your daily life. Here are some recommendations for tailoring your daily routine to Kapha dosha:

Wake up early, ideally before sunrise.

Drink warm water with lemon and honey in the morning to help stimulate digestion and metabolism.

Eat light, warming foods such as spicy soups, ginger tea, or steamed vegetables.

Practice invigorating yoga or other forms of exercise such as running or dancing.

Incorporate stimulating activities such as learning a new skill, trying a new hobby, or socializing with friends.

Use stimulating essential oils such as eucalyptus, rosemary, or grapefruit.

Avoid overeating or indulging in heavy, oily foods.

Benefits of Tailoring Your Daily Routine to Your Dosha:

1. Promotes balance and harmony: Tailoring your daily routine to your dosha can help promote balance and harmony within your body, mind, and spirit.

2. Enhances energy and vitality: By understanding your dosha, you can make choices in your daily routine that support your individual needs and promote optimal energy and vitality.

3. Reduces stress and promotes relaxation: Tailoring your routine to your dosha can help

Ayurvedic Yoga and Exercise

Ayurvedic yoga and exercise are an important part of Ayurvedic medicine and can help promote optimal health and wellbeing. By combining the principles of Ayurveda with yoga and exercise, individuals can create a personalized routine that supports their unique dosha and promotes balance and harmony within the body and mind.

The Principles of Ayurvedic Yoga and Exercise:

Ayurvedic yoga and exercise are based on the principles of the doshas, which are the three biological energies that govern the body and mind. Each dosha has unique characteristics and tendencies, and by understanding your dosha, you can choose yoga and exercise practices that support your individual needs.

Vata Dosha:

If you have a predominant Vata dosha, you may be naturally creative, energetic, and adaptable, but may also be prone to anxiety, worry, and nervousness. To balance Vata dosha through yoga and exercise, it is important to focus on grounding and stabilizing practices, such as:

Hatha yoga, which emphasizes slow, gentle movements and breathwork.

Restorative yoga, which involves supported postures and relaxation techniques.

Tai Chi or Qi Gong, which incorporate gentle, flowing movements and meditation.

Walking or other low-impact exercises that promote circulation and grounding.

Incorporating deep breathing exercises such as pranayama into your practice.

Pitta Dosha:

If you have a predominant Pitta dosha, you may be naturally confident, organized, and focused, but may also be prone to irritability, anger, and inflammation. To balance Pitta dosha through yoga and exercise, it is important to focus on calming and cooling practices, such as:

Yin yoga, which involves long-held poses and focuses on connective tissues and joints.

Yoga nidra, which involves guided meditation and deep relaxation.

Swimming or other water-based exercises that promote cooling and relaxation.

Incorporating cooling pranayama exercises such as Sheetali or Sheetkari into your practice.

Avoiding high-intensity or competitive exercises that can increase Pitta dosha.

Kapha Dosha:

If you have a predominant Kapha dosha, you may be naturally calm, grounded, and nurturing, but may also be prone to lethargy, weight gain, and stagnation. To balance Kapha dosha through yoga and exercise, it is important to focus on stimulating and invigorating practices, such as:

Power yoga or vinyasa flow, which involves fast-paced movements and breathwork.

Kundalini yoga, which incorporates dynamic movements, breathwork, and meditation.

Cardiovascular exercises such as running or cycling.

Incorporating stimulating pranayama exercises such as Bhastrika or Kapalbhati into your practice.

Avoiding sedentary or repetitive exercises that can increase Kapha dosha.

Benefits of Ayurvedic Yoga and Exercise:

1. Promotes balance and harmony: Ayurvedic yoga and exercise can help promote balance and harmony within the body and mind by tailoring practices to your unique dosha.

2. Enhances energy and vitality: By choosing yoga and exercise practices that support your individual needs, you can promote optimal energy and vitality.

3. Reduces stress and promotes relaxation: Yoga and exercise practices that focus on relaxation and grounding can help reduce stress and promote relaxation.

4. Increases strength and flexibility: Yoga and exercise practices can increase strength, flexibility, and overall physical fitness.

5. Promotes self-awareness: By practicing Ayurvedic yoga and exercise, you can increase self-awareness and develop a deeper understanding of your body and mind.

Incorporating Ayurvedic yoga and exercise practices into your daily routine can be a powerful way to

Yoga's connection to Ayurveda

Yoga and Ayurveda are sister sciences that have been practiced together for thousands of years in India. Both practices seek to promote physical, mental, and spiritual wellbeing, and share a common understanding of the body, mind, and consciousness.

Yoga and Ayurveda share many similarities in their philosophies and practices. Both systems recognize that the body, mind, and spirit are interconnected and that maintaining balance and harmony within these aspects of our being is essential for optimal health and wellbeing. Additionally, both practices are rooted in ancient Vedic texts, which emphasize the importance of a holistic approach to health and wellbeing.

Ayurveda and Yoga's Shared Principles:

The principles of Ayurveda and Yoga overlap in many ways. Some of these shared principles include:

1. The Three Doshas: Ayurveda recognizes three doshas or biological energies that govern the body and mind, while Yoga recognizes three gunas or qualities that determine a person's character and actions.

2. The Importance of Breath: Both practices emphasize the importance of breath in promoting physical, mental, and spiritual health.

3. The Concept of Prana: Ayurveda and Yoga both recognize the concept of prana or life force energy, which flows through the body and can be manipulated through practices such as pranayama and Ayurvedic treatments.

4. The Importance of Meditation: Both practices recognize the importance of meditation in promoting mental and spiritual wellbeing.

5. The Role of Diet and Lifestyle: Ayurveda and Yoga both recognize the role of diet and lifestyle in promoting optimal health and wellbeing.

Ayurveda and Yoga's Complementary Practices:

Ayurveda and Yoga also have complementary practices that can enhance each other's benefits. For example:

6. Yoga can help balance the doshas: By practicing yoga postures and breathing exercises that are tailored to your dosha, you can help balance the doshas and promote overall health and wellbeing.

7. Ayurveda can support yoga practice: Ayurvedic treatments such as massages, oil treatments, and herbal supplements can help support a yoga practice by promoting physical and mental relaxation and reducing stress.

8. Ayurvedic diet can enhance yoga practice: Eating a diet that is tailored to your dosha can help support a yoga practice by providing the body with the nutrients it needs for optimal performance.

9. Yoga can deepen meditation practice: By incorporating yoga postures and breathing exercises into your meditation practice, you can deepen your meditation and promote mental and spiritual wellbeing.

Benefits of Combining Ayurveda and Yoga:

10. Promotes physical, mental, and spiritual wellbeing: By combining Ayurveda and Yoga practices, you can promote overall physical, mental, and spiritual health and wellbeing.

11. Supports individual needs: By tailoring Ayurvedic treatments and yoga practices to your individual dosha and needs, you can create a personalized approach to health and wellbeing.

12. Enhances self-awareness: By practicing Ayurveda and Yoga together, you can increase self-awareness and develop a deeper understanding of your body, mind, and consciousness.

13. Reduces stress and promotes relaxation: Both Ayurveda and Yoga practices can help reduce stress and promote relaxation, leading to improved overall wellbeing.

14. Increases energy and vitality: Ayurveda and Yoga practices can help increase energy and vitality, leading to improved physical, mental, and spiritual performance.

Dosha-specific yoga poses and sequences

1. Ayurveda and Yoga are sister sciences that have been practiced together for thousands of years in India. Ayurveda recognizes three doshas or biological energies that govern the body and mind: Vata, Pitta, and Kapha. Each dosha has unique physical and mental characteristics, and therefore requires a specific approach to yoga practice.

Vata Dosha:

Vata is the principle of movement and governs all bodily functions related to movement, such as breathing, circulation, and digestion. People with a predominant Vata dosha tend to have a thin body frame, dry skin, and a restless and creative mind. They also tend to experience anxiety, nervousness, and insomnia.

Yoga poses and sequences for Vata:

2. Sun Salutations: Sun Salutations are a great way to warm up the body and increase circulation, which is important for people with a Vata constitution who tend to have cold hands and feet.

3. Forward Folds: Forward folds help to calm the mind and release tension in the body, which is beneficial for people with a Vata constitution who tend to be anxious and restless.

4. Standing Poses: Standing poses help to ground the body and promote stability, which is important for people with a Vata constitution who tend to be ungrounded and flighty.

5. Twists: Twists help to stimulate digestion and promote the elimination of waste, which is important for people with a Vata constitution who tend to have irregular digestion.

6. Restorative Poses: Restorative poses help to promote deep relaxation and release tension in the body, which is beneficial for people with a Vata constitution who tend to experience anxiety and insomnia.

Pitta Dosha:

Pitta is the principle of transformation and governs all bodily functions related to digestion, metabolism, and energy production. People with a predominant Pitta dosha tend to have a medium build, oily skin, and a sharp intellect. They also tend to experience anger, irritability, and frustration.

Yoga poses and sequences for Pitta:

7. Cooling Poses: Cooling poses such as forward folds and gentle twists help to balance Pitta's tendency towards heat and inflammation.

8. Chest Openers: Chest openers help to release tension in the chest and promote deep breathing, which is beneficial for people with a Pitta constitution who tend to hold tension in the chest and have shallow breathing.

9. Inversions: Inversions help to calm the mind and promote relaxation, which is beneficial for people with a Pitta constitution who tend to experience anger and frustration.

10. Backbends: Backbends help to energize the body and promote a positive outlook, which is important for people with a Pitta constitution who tend to be overly critical and judgmental.

11. Restorative Poses: Restorative poses help to promote deep relaxation and release tension in the body, which is beneficial for people with a Pitta constitution who tend to experience stress and anxiety.

Kapha Dosha:

Kapha is the principle of structure and stability and governs all bodily functions related to structure, such as bone density and muscle mass. People with a predominant Kapha dosha tend to have a heavy body frame, oily skin, and a calm and steady mind. They also tend to experience lethargy, dullness, and depression.

Yoga poses and sequences for Kapha:

12. Energizing Poses: Energizing poses such as Sun Salutations and inversions help to stimulate the body and promote energy flow, which is important for people with a Kapha constitution who tend to feel lethargic.

13. Standing Poses: Standing poses help to promote stability and balance, which is important for people with a Kapha constitution who tend to have a heavy body frame.

3

Ayurvedic guidelines for physical activity

Ayurveda recognizes the importance of physical activity for overall health and well-being. However, the type and amount of physical activity recommended varies according to each person's dosha or biological energy.

Vata Dosha:

People with a Vata constitution tend to have a high level of physical activity and energy, but they can easily become overstimulated or fatigued. Therefore, it's important for people with a Vata constitution to engage in activities that are grounding, calming, and promote stability. Some recommendations include:

1. Yoga: Yoga is an ideal physical activity for people with a Vata constitution because it promotes relaxation, grounding, and balance.

2. Walking: Walking is a low-impact activity that helps to promote circulation and grounding, which is important for people with a Vata constitution who tend to have cold hands and feet.

3. Tai Chi: Tai Chi is a gentle form of exercise that promotes balance and relaxation, which is beneficial for people with a Vata constitution who tend to be anxious and restless.

4. Dancing: Dancing is a fun and energizing activity that helps to promote movement and creativity, which is important for people with a Vata constitution who tend to be creative and imaginative.

Pitta Dosha:

People with a Pitta constitution tend to have a high level of physical activity and energy, but they can easily become overheated or exhausted. Therefore, it's important for people with a Pitta constitution to engage in activities that are cooling, calming, and promote relaxation. Some recommendations include:

5. Swimming: Swimming is a great physical activity for people with a Pitta constitution because it promotes cooling and relaxation.

6. Hiking: Hiking is a low-impact activity that promotes a connection to nature and grounding, which is important for people with a Pitta constitution who tend to be focused on achievement and productivity.

7. Biking: Biking is an energizing activity that promotes movement and fun, which is important for people with a Pitta constitution who tend to be competitive and driven.

8. Yoga: Yoga is a beneficial physical activity for people with a Pitta constitution because it promotes cooling and relaxation.

Kapha Dosha:

People with a Kapha constitution tend to have a lower level of physical activity and energy, but they can easily become sluggish or stagnant. Therefore, it's important for people with a Kapha constitution to engage in activities that are energizing, stimulating, and promote movement. Some recommendations include:

9. Cardiovascular exercise: Cardiovascular exercise such as running or aerobics is an ideal physical activity for people with a Kapha constitution because it promotes energy and movement.

10. Weight training: Weight training is a beneficial physical activity for people with a Kapha constitution because it promotes muscle strength and energy.

11. Dancing: Dancing is a fun and energizing activity that helps to promote movement and creativity, which is important for people with a Kapha constitution who tend to be sluggish.

12. Yoga: Yoga is a beneficial physical activity for people with a Kapha constitution because it promotes movement and energy.

In general, Ayurveda recommends that physical activity should be done in moderation and should be tailored to each person's individual needs and dosha. It's important to listen to your body and not push yourself too hard, as this can lead to imbalances and health issues. Additionally, Ayurveda emphasizes the importance of warm-up and cool-down periods before and after physical activity to prevent injury and promote recovery.

Ayurvedic Stress Management

Stress is a common problem in modern life, and it can have a negative impact on both physical and mental health. In Ayurveda, stress is viewed as an imbalance in the doshas, and there are many effective strategies for managing stress and promoting relaxation.

Understanding Stress in Ayurveda:

According to Ayurveda, stress is caused by an imbalance in the doshas, specifically an excess of Vata or Pitta. Vata imbalances can lead to anxiety, fear, and worry, while Pitta imbalances can cause anger, irritability, and frustration.

Stress can also lead to imbalances in the body, such as high blood pressure, insomnia, and digestive issues. Therefore, it's important to address stress at both the physical and mental levels in order to promote overall health and well-being.

Ayurvedic Stress Management Techniques:

1. Meditation: Meditation is a powerful tool for managing stress in Ayurveda. Regular meditation practice can help to calm the mind, reduce anxiety, and promote relaxation.

2. Pranayama: Pranayama, or yogic breathing techniques, can be used to reduce stress and promote relaxation. Techniques such as alternate nostril breathing and deep breathing can help to calm the mind and balance the doshas.

3. Yoga: Yoga is a holistic practice that can help to reduce stress and promote relaxation. Gentle yoga poses such as forward bends and child's pose can be especially helpful for reducing anxiety and promoting relaxation.

4. Massage: Ayurvedic massage, also known as Abhyanga, can be used to reduce stress and promote relaxation. Massage helps to increase circulation and release tension in the muscles, which can help to promote relaxation and reduce stress.

5. Herbal Remedies: Ayurveda offers a variety of herbal remedies that can help to reduce stress and promote relaxation. Ashwagandha is an adaptogenic herb that can help to reduce anxiety and promote relaxation, while Brahmi can help to improve memory and cognitive function.

6. Aromatherapy: Essential oils can be used in aromatherapy to reduce stress and promote relaxation. Lavender, chamomile, and bergamot are all popular essential oils for reducing stress and promoting relaxation.

7. Diet and Lifestyle: Ayurveda emphasizes the importance of a healthy diet and lifestyle for managing stress. Eating a balanced diet that is tailored to your dosha can help to promote overall health and well-being, while engaging in regular physical activity can help to reduce stress and promote relaxation.

In addition to these techniques, it's important to address the root cause of stress and make any necessary lifestyle changes. This may include reducing work hours, practicing better time management, and engaging in self-care activities such as meditation, yoga, and massage.

The impact of stress on the doshas

In Ayurveda, the ancient system of medicine from India, the doshas are the three primary forces that govern the physical and mental characteristics of a person. The three doshas are Vata, Pitta, and Kapha, and they are responsible for various bodily functions, including digestion, metabolism, and mental and emotional states. When these doshas are in balance, a person experiences good health and well-being. However, when there is an imbalance, it can lead to various health problems, including stress.

Stress is a common problem in modern society, and it can have a significant impact on the doshas. According to Ayurveda, stress is caused by an imbalance in the doshas, specifically an excess of Vata or Pitta. Vata imbalances can lead to anxiety, fear, and worry, while Pitta imbalances can cause anger, irritability, and frustration.

The impact of stress on the doshas can be seen in various ways. Here are some of the ways in which stress can affect the different doshas:

1. Vata: Vata is the dosha that governs movement and is responsible for functions such as breathing, circulation, and nervous system activity. When Vata is imbalanced due to stress, it can lead to anxiety, restlessness, insomnia, and digestive problems such as bloating and constipation. Vata imbalances can also cause joint pain, dry skin, and cold hands and feet.

2. Pitta: Pitta is the dosha that governs transformation and is responsible for functions such as digestion, metabolism, and hormone production. When Pitta is imbalanced due to stress, it can lead to anger, irritability, and frustration. It can also cause digestive problems such as acid reflux, diarrhea, and inflammation in the body.

3. Kapha: Kapha is the dosha that governs structure and stability and is responsible for functions such as immunity, strength, and lubrication. When Kapha is imbalanced due to stress, it can lead to lethargy, depression, and weight gain. Kapha imbalances can also cause respiratory problems such as allergies and congestion.

It's important to note that stress can affect all three doshas, but the type of stress and the individual's constitution will determine which dosha is most affected. For example, a person with a Vata constitution may be more prone to anxiety and insomnia when stressed, while a person with a Pitta constitution may be more prone to anger and digestive problems.

In Ayurveda, it's essential to address stress at the root cause and not just treat the symptoms. This may include making lifestyle changes, engaging in stress-reducing activities such as meditation and yoga, and using herbs and other natural remedies to balance the doshas.

Some of the Ayurvedic herbs that can help to balance the doshas and reduce stress include Ashwagandha, Brahmi, and Shatavari. Ashwagandha is an adaptogenic herb that can help to reduce anxiety and promote relaxation, while Brahmi can help to improve memory and cognitive function. Shatavari is a nourishing herb that can help to balance the hormones and support overall health and well-being.

In addition to herbal remedies, lifestyle changes can also be effective in reducing stress and balancing the doshas. Ayurveda recommends following a daily routine, known as dinacharya, which includes practices such as waking up early, meditation, and exercise. It's also important to follow a balanced diet that is tailored to your dosha and to engage in self-care activities such as massage and aromatherapy.

Ayurvedic techniques for managing stress

Ayurveda is a holistic system of medicine that has been practiced in India for over 5,000 years. It offers a variety of techniques for managing stress, which is a significant health issue in today's world. Ayurvedic stress management techniques are designed to restore balance to the mind and body, and to promote overall health and well-being.

One of the primary ways that Ayurveda manages stress is through the use of herbs and spices. Many Ayurvedic herbs have been shown to have a calming effect on the body and mind, including ashwagandha, brahmi, and jatamansi. These herbs can be taken in supplement form, or used in cooking to add flavor and health benefits to meals.

Another important aspect of Ayurvedic stress management is the practice of yoga and meditation. These practices have been shown to reduce stress and anxiety, and to promote feelings of relaxation and well-being. In Ayurveda, yoga and meditation are tailored to the individual's dosha, or constitution, to ensure that the practice is most effective for their unique needs.

Massage is another Ayurvedic technique for managing stress. Ayurvedic massage, or abhyanga, uses warm oils and gentle pressure to promote relaxation and rejuvenation. This technique can be especially effective for those who carry tension in their muscles, and can help to release built-up stress and tension in the body.

Diet and lifestyle modifications are also an important part of Ayurvedic stress management. Eating a balanced diet of whole, fresh foods can help to nourish the body and promote overall health. Additionally, practicing good sleep hygiene, such as avoiding screens before bedtime and establishing a regular sleep routine, can help to reduce stress and promote restful sleep.

Ayurveda also emphasizes the importance of self-care and taking time to prioritize one's own well-being. This can include activities such as taking a relaxing bath, spending time in nature, or practicing a hobby that brings joy and relaxation.

In Ayurveda, it is believed that stress and anxiety are often caused by an imbalance in the doshas. Therefore, Ayurvedic stress management techniques are designed to restore balance to the body and mind, and to promote overall health and well-being. By taking a holistic approach to stress management, Ayurveda offers a unique and effective way to reduce stress and promote optimal health.

Meditation and mindfulness in Ayurveda

Meditation and mindfulness have been a fundamental part of Ayurvedic practice for thousands of years. These techniques are designed to promote relaxation, reduce stress, and cultivate a sense of inner peace and well-being. In Ayurveda, meditation and mindfulness are considered essential practices for balancing the mind and body, and promoting optimal health and vitality.

Meditation is a practice that involves training the mind to focus and become more aware of the present moment. In Ayurveda, meditation is used to cultivate a sense of inner calm, improve mental clarity and focus, and reduce stress and anxiety. There are many different types of meditation techniques, but some of the most common ones in Ayurveda include mindfulness meditation, mantra meditation, and breath awareness meditation.

Mindfulness is a related practice that involves paying attention to the present moment without judgment. This practice can help to reduce stress and anxiety, improve mental clarity and focus, and promote a sense of inner peace and well-being. Mindfulness can be practiced in many different ways, such as through meditation, mindful breathing, or mindful movement.

In Ayurveda, meditation and mindfulness are often tailored to the individual's dosha, or constitution. This helps to ensure that the practice is most effective for the individual's unique needs. For example, those with a Vata constitution may benefit from meditation practices that are grounding and calming, while those with a Pitta constitution may benefit from practices that are cooling and calming.

Meditation and mindfulness can be practiced in many different settings and situations. Some people prefer to practice in a quiet, secluded space, while others find it helpful to incorporate mindfulness into their daily activities, such as cooking or walking. There are also many resources available for those who want to learn more about meditation and mindfulness, including books, classes, and online resources.

In addition to promoting relaxation and reducing stress, meditation and mindfulness have also been shown to have a variety of health benefits. Studies have shown that these practices can help to lower blood pressure, reduce symptoms of depression and anxiety, and improve immune function. They may also be helpful for managing chronic pain and other health conditions.

Ayurveda also emphasizes the importance of incorporating mindfulness into daily activities, such as eating and exercise. This can help to promote greater awareness of the body and its needs, and can lead to healthier lifestyle habits overall. For example, practicing mindful eating can help to promote greater satisfaction with food, reduce overeating, and improve digestion.

Ayurvedic Sleep and Rest

Sleep and rest are essential components of Ayurvedic practice. Adequate rest and sleep are necessary for maintaining optimal health and well-being, as they help to restore and rejuvenate the body and mind. In Ayurveda, sleep is considered one of the three pillars of health, along with diet and lifestyle.

Ayurveda recognizes that different individuals have different sleep needs based on their dosha. Vata types tend to need more sleep than Pitta or Kapha types, while Pitta types may have trouble falling asleep due to their active minds, and Kapha types may have trouble waking up due to their tendency towards lethargy. By understanding these differences, Ayurveda offers a range of techniques and practices to help individuals of all doshas achieve restful, rejuvenating sleep.

One of the key Ayurvedic practices for promoting restful sleep is establishing a regular sleep routine. This involves going to bed and waking up at the same time each day, which helps to regulate the body's natural sleep-wake cycle. It is also important to create a relaxing sleep environment, free from distractions and excess stimulation. This might include things like minimizing screen time before bed, creating a comfortable sleep space, and using calming scents or sounds to promote relaxation.

Ayurveda also emphasizes the importance of winding down before bed. This might involve practicing gentle yoga or meditation, taking a warm bath, or engaging in other relaxing activities that help to quiet the mind and promote a sense of calm. It is also important to avoid stimulating activities before bed, such as intense exercise or work-related tasks, which can interfere with the body's ability to relax and fall asleep.

In addition to establishing healthy sleep habits, Ayurveda also recommends a number of natural remedies for promoting restful sleep. These might include things like drinking herbal teas, such as chamomile or valerian root, using aromatherapy oils like lavender or sandalwood, or taking natural supplements like melatonin or magnesium. It is important to consult with a qualified Ayurvedic practitioner before beginning any new supplement or herbal remedy, to ensure that it is safe and appropriate for your individual needs.

Ayurveda also recognizes the importance of rest and relaxation throughout the day. In addition to getting adequate sleep at night, it is important to take breaks and allow the body and mind to rest and recharge throughout the day. This might involve taking short breaks during work or study to stretch, meditate, or simply rest the eyes, or incorporating restful activities like gentle yoga or tai chi into the daily routine.

The importance of sleep in Ayurveda

Ayurveda, the ancient Indian system of medicine, places great emphasis on sleep as an essential component of health and wellbeing. According to Ayurveda, sleep is not merely a state of inactivity or rest, but a dynamic process of rejuvenation that allows the body and mind to heal and repair.

In Ayurveda, sleep is closely linked to the three doshas – Vata, Pitta, and Kapha – and imbalances in these doshas can lead to sleep disturbances and disorders. For example, excess Vata can cause restlessness and anxiety, Pitta imbalance can result in insomnia and waking up feeling hot and irritable, while Kapha imbalance can lead to excessive sleep and difficulty waking up in the morning.

Ayurveda also recognizes the importance of circadian rhythms, the natural biological rhythms that govern our sleep-wake cycles. According to Ayurveda, our bodies are naturally attuned to the cycles of the sun and moon, and sleep during the nighttime hours is considered most beneficial for health and wellbeing.

To promote restful and rejuvenating sleep, Ayurveda recommends a variety of practices and lifestyle changes. Here are some of the key Ayurvedic principles and techniques for promoting healthy sleep:

1. Stick to a regular sleep schedule: Ayurveda emphasizes the importance of going to bed and waking up at the same time every day. This helps regulate the body's circadian rhythms and can improve the quality of sleep.

2. Create a calming bedtime routine: Establishing a relaxing bedtime routine can help signal to the body that it's time for sleep. This might include taking a warm bath, practicing gentle yoga or meditation, or drinking a cup of warm herbal tea.

3. Avoid stimulating activities before bed: In order to promote restful sleep, Ayurveda recommends avoiding stimulating activities in the hours leading up to bedtime. This might include watching TV or using electronic devices, engaging in heated arguments, or engaging in strenuous exercise.

4. Create a comfortable sleep environment: The physical environment in which we sleep can have a significant impact on the quality of our sleep. Ayurveda recommends creating a cool, dark, and quiet sleep environment, free from distractions and disruptions.

5. Follow an Ayurvedic diet: The foods we eat can also have an impact on the quality of our sleep. Following an Ayurvedic diet, which emphasizes fresh, whole foods and avoids processed and refined foods, can help promote restful sleep.

6. Practice relaxation techniques: Ayurveda recommends a variety of relaxation techniques to help promote restful sleep, including yoga, meditation, and pranayama (breathing exercises).

7. Use natural remedies: Ayurveda also employs a variety of natural remedies to promote restful sleep, including herbal teas, aromatherapy, and Ayurvedic herbs and supplements.

By following these Ayurvedic principles and techniques, individuals can promote restful, rejuvenating sleep and support overall health and wellbeing. As with all aspects of Ayurveda, it's important to work with a qualified Ayurvedic practitioner to determine the best approach for your individual needs and circumstances.

Ayurvedic guidelines for quality sleep

Ayurveda is a holistic system of health and wellness that originated in ancient India over 5000 years ago. One of the pillars of Ayurveda is the importance of proper sleep and rest for maintaining good health. In Ayurveda, sleep is seen as essential for the body to rest and repair itself, and for the mind to process and integrate experiences.

According to Ayurveda, sleep is regulated by the doshas - Vata, Pitta, and Kapha - and imbalances in these doshas can lead to sleep disturbances and insomnia. Therefore, understanding your individual dosha and balancing it through diet, lifestyle, and herbal remedies can help promote restful sleep.

The Ayurvedic approach to sleep is not only focused on the duration of sleep, but also on the quality of sleep. It is believed that the body is most receptive to healing during the hours of 10 pm to 2 am, and that deep, uninterrupted sleep during this time is crucial for optimal health. Here are some Ayurvedic guidelines for quality sleep:

1. Establish a regular sleep routine: Going to bed and waking up at the same time every day helps regulate the body's natural sleep-wake cycle, or circadian rhythm. This can help promote deeper, more restful sleep.

2. Create a relaxing sleep environment: The bedroom should be a peaceful and calming space. Keeping the room dark, cool, and free from electronic devices can help promote better sleep. Additionally, incorporating relaxing scents like lavender or chamomile can help soothe the mind and promote relaxation.

3. Avoid stimulating activities before bedtime: Engaging in stimulating activities like watching TV, using electronic devices, or engaging in intense exercise before bedtime can disrupt the body's natural sleep-wake cycle and make it harder to fall asleep.

4. Incorporate relaxing activities before bedtime: Engaging in relaxing activities before bedtime can help promote a sense of calm and relaxation. This could include gentle yoga, meditation, reading a book, or taking a warm bath.

5. Follow an appropriate diet: Eating heavy, spicy, or greasy foods before bedtime can make it harder to fall asleep and lead to indigestion. Instead, opt for lighter, nourishing foods that are easier to digest.

6. Use herbs and supplements: Certain herbs and supplements, such as ashwagandha, brahmi, and valerian root, can help promote relaxation and restful sleep. However, it is important to consult with a qualified Ayurvedic practitioner before using any herbs or supplements.

7. Practice self-care: Engaging in self-care practices like Abhyanga (Ayurvedic self-massage) or Shirodhara (a therapeutic Ayurvedic treatment where a continuous stream of warm oil is poured over the forehead) can help promote relaxation and improve sleep quality.

Dosha-specific sleep recommendations

Ayurveda, the ancient Indian system of medicine, recognizes the importance of quality sleep for overall health and wellbeing. According to Ayurveda, sleep is a vital component in balancing the doshas, and a lack of quality sleep can lead to imbalances and health issues. Therefore, Ayurveda offers dosha-specific sleep recommendations to ensure restful and rejuvenating sleep.

Vata Dosha and Sleep

People with a predominance of Vata dosha tend to have a more irregular sleep pattern, which can lead to difficulty falling asleep or staying asleep. Therefore, it is essential for Vata types to follow a consistent sleep routine to promote quality sleep. Some tips for Vata sleep include:

1. Stick to a consistent sleep schedule: Try to go to bed and wake up at the same time every day, even on weekends.

2. Wind-down routine: Establish a relaxing pre-sleep routine, such as taking a warm bath or practicing relaxation techniques like yoga or meditation.

3. Avoid stimulating activities: Avoid stimulating activities like working on the computer or watching TV before bed, as these can interfere with the ability to fall asleep.

4. Create a cozy sleep environment: Ensure the sleeping area is warm, quiet, and comfortable, as Vata types tend to be more sensitive to cold temperatures and noise.

Pitta Dosha and Sleep

People with a predominance of Pitta dosha tend to have a more intense and driven nature, which can cause difficulty in falling asleep due to an overactive mind. Therefore, it is essential for Pitta types to engage in relaxing activities before bed to promote quality sleep. Some tips for Pitta sleep include:

5. Establish a regular sleep routine: Similar to Vata, it is essential for Pitta types to stick to a consistent sleep schedule to promote quality sleep.

6. Limit stimulating activities: Avoid engaging in stimulating activities before bed, like exercising or working on the computer, as these can lead to an overactive mind and difficulty falling asleep.

7. Relaxing activities: Practice relaxation techniques like deep breathing exercises or meditation to calm the mind and promote relaxation.

8. Create a cool sleep environment: Ensure the sleeping area is cool and comfortable, as Pitta types tend to be more sensitive to heat and humidity.

Kapha Dosha and Sleep

People with a predominance of Kapha dosha tend to have a more relaxed and calm nature, which can lead to excessive sleep and difficulty waking up in the morning. Therefore, it is essential for Kapha types to engage in stimulating activities to promote quality sleep and wakefulness. Some tips for Kapha sleep include:

9. Establish a consistent sleep routine: Similar to Vata and Pitta, it is essential for Kapha types to stick to a consistent sleep schedule to promote quality sleep.

10. Engage in stimulating activities: Engage in stimulating activities before bed, such as a light workout or reading a stimulating book, to promote wakefulness and quality sleep.

11. Avoid excessive sleep: Avoid oversleeping, as this can lead to lethargy and a feeling of heaviness upon waking up.

12. Create a bright sleep environment: Ensure the sleeping area is bright and airy, as Kapha types tend to be more prone to feeling heavy and stagnant.

Ayurvedic Skincare and Beauty

Ayurveda, an ancient system of medicine from India, emphasizes the importance of maintaining overall well-being through a balanced lifestyle, including skincare and beauty practices. According to Ayurveda, beauty and radiance come from within, and external factors such as the environment and diet play a significant role in skin health. Therefore, Ayurvedic skincare and beauty practices focus on nourishing the body and mind from the inside out.

Ayurveda recognizes three doshas, or constitutions, which influence individual physical, mental, and emotional traits. Each dosha has specific characteristics that affect skin health and beauty. Understanding one's dosha can help identify the best skincare practices to maintain healthy, radiant skin.

Vata skin is dry, thin, and delicate, with a tendency towards wrinkles, fine lines, and dark circles. Pitta skin is sensitive, prone to redness, and has a tendency towards acne, rosacea, and sunspots. Kapha skin is thick, oily, and prone to enlarged pores, blackheads, and pimples.

Ayurvedic skincare and beauty practices aim to balance the doshas and promote overall skin health. Here are some of the Ayurvedic skincare and beauty practices:

1. Cleansing: Ayurveda emphasizes the importance of cleansing the skin to remove impurities and maintain skin health. Cleansing also helps to balance the doshas and prepare the skin for further treatment. Ayurvedic cleansers include natural ingredients like honey, milk, and turmeric, which have anti-inflammatory and antibacterial properties.

2. Exfoliating: Exfoliating removes dead skin cells and stimulates the production of new skin cells, promoting a more youthful and radiant complexion. Ayurvedic exfoliants use natural ingredients like powdered herbs, lentils, and grains, which gently remove impurities without stripping the skin of its natural oils.

3. Moisturizing: Ayurvedic moisturizers use natural ingredients like ghee, coconut oil, and almond oil, which nourish and hydrate the skin without clogging pores. Moisturizing helps to balance the doshas and prevent dryness, which can lead to premature aging.

4. Massage: Ayurvedic facial massage stimulates blood flow and lymphatic drainage, promoting the elimination of toxins and impurities. Massage also helps to relax facial muscles and reduce the appearance of fine lines and wrinkles. Ayurvedic massage oils include sesame oil, almond oil, and coconut oil, which have nourishing and hydrating properties.

5. Herbal remedies: Ayurveda uses herbal remedies to treat specific skin concerns, such as acne, rosacea, and hyperpigmentation. Ayurvedic herbs like neem, turmeric, and aloe vera have antibacterial and anti-inflammatory properties, which help to soothe and heal the skin.

6. Diet and lifestyle: Ayurvedic skincare and beauty practices also include dietary and lifestyle recommendations. Eating a healthy, balanced diet that includes fresh fruits and vegetables, whole grains, and lean protein can help to nourish the skin from the inside out. Getting enough sleep, managing stress, and practicing self-care can also promote healthy, radiant skin.

Ayurvedic skincare principles

Ayurveda, the ancient Indian system of healing, emphasizes the importance of maintaining harmony between the mind, body, and spirit. One way to achieve this balance is through proper skincare. Ayurvedic skincare principles focus on using natural ingredients, personalized routines, and self-care practices to achieve healthy and glowing skin.

According to Ayurveda, skin reflects a person's internal health and well-being. Imbalances in the doshas can manifest as skin problems such as acne, dryness, or inflammation. Therefore, Ayurvedic skincare aims to restore balance and promote overall health.

One of the foundational principles of Ayurvedic skincare is using natural ingredients. Ayurvedic texts mention various herbs, oils, and other natural substances that can benefit the skin. For instance, aloe vera is a cooling and soothing herb that can alleviate inflammation and redness. Neem, known as the "village pharmacy" in India, has antibacterial and antifungal properties that can help treat acne and other skin conditions. Turmeric is a potent antioxidant that can brighten the skin and reduce signs of aging.

In Ayurveda, skincare routines are personalized based on a person's dosha. For instance, those with a Pitta dosha tend to have sensitive skin that is prone to inflammation and sunburn. Therefore, their skincare routine should focus on cooling and soothing the skin. Those with a Vata dosha tend to have dry skin, so their skincare routine should focus on moisturization and nourishment. Those with a Kapha dosha tend to have oily skin that is prone to congestion, so their skincare routine should focus on cleansing and exfoliation.

Ayurvedic skincare also emphasizes the importance of self-care practices such as meditation, pranayama (breathing exercises), and yoga. These practices can help reduce stress, improve circulation, and promote overall well-being, which can translate to healthier skin.

Another aspect of Ayurvedic skincare is paying attention to the seasons and adjusting skincare routines accordingly. In Ayurveda, each season is associated with a dosha. For instance, the summer season is associated with Pitta dosha, and excess heat and sun exposure can aggravate Pitta imbalances in the body and skin. Therefore, during the summer, it is recommended to use cooling and soothing skincare products, wear protective clothing and hats, and avoid excess sun exposure.

Dosha-specific skincare recommendations

Ayurveda, the ancient Indian system of medicine, recognizes that each person is unique and has a distinct constitution, or dosha. Understanding your dosha is an important first step in creating a personalized skincare routine that addresses your individual needs. Below we will discuss the dosha-specific skincare recommendations in Ayurveda.

Vata skin tends to be dry, thin, and delicate. It is prone to fine lines, wrinkles, and premature aging. To balance vata skin, it is important to use nourishing, hydrating, and grounding skincare products. Oils like sesame, almond, and jojoba are excellent for moisturizing vata skin. Other nourishing ingredients include ghee, honey, and avocado. Vata skin should also be protected from the sun and wind, as these elements can aggravate dryness and sensitivity. A gentle facial massage with warm oil can help to improve circulation and bring a healthy glow to vata skin.

Pitta skin is characterized by sensitivity, redness, and inflammation. It is prone to acne, rosacea, and other inflammatory skin conditions. To balance pitta skin, it is important to use cooling, soothing, and anti-inflammatory skincare products. Aloe vera, cucumber, and chamomile are excellent ingredients for pitta skin. Rose water can be used as a toner to reduce inflammation and redness. Pitta skin should be protected from the sun, as it is more prone to sunburn and heat rash. A cool compress or aloe vera gel can be used to soothe and calm irritated pitta skin.

Kapha skin tends to be oily, thick, and congested. It is prone to blackheads, whiteheads, and acne. To balance kapha skin, it is important to use cleansing, detoxifying, and stimulating skincare products. Clay masks, exfoliants, and astringent toners are excellent for kapha skin. Ingredients like lemon, grapefruit, and ginger can help to detoxify and stimulate the skin. Kapha skin should be protected from excessive moisture, as this can aggravate oiliness and congestion. Regular exercise and a healthy diet can also help to balance kapha skin.

In addition to using dosha-specific skincare products, Ayurveda emphasizes the importance of a healthy lifestyle for beautiful, radiant skin. Eating a balanced diet, staying hydrated, getting regular exercise, and managing stress are all important factors in maintaining healthy skin. Ayurvedic practices like oil pulling and dry brushing can also help to detoxify the body and promote healthy skin.

Ayurvedic beauty rituals and treatments

Ayurveda, the ancient Indian system of medicine, emphasizes a holistic approach to health and beauty. According to Ayurveda, beauty is not just skin-deep but is a reflection of overall health and wellbeing. Ayurvedic beauty rituals and treatments are designed to help maintain a healthy balance of the doshas, nourish the skin, and enhance natural beauty. Below we will explore some of the most popular Ayurvedic beauty rituals and treatments and their benefits.

Oil Massage (Abhyanga)

Abhyanga is an Ayurvedic full-body massage that involves the use of warm herbal oils. The massage is performed in a specific sequence to stimulate the marma points, which are vital energy centers in the body. Abhyanga helps to nourish and rejuvenate the skin, reduce stress, promote relaxation, and balance the doshas. The type of oil used for the massage may vary based on the individual's dosha. For example, Vata individuals may benefit from warming oils such as sesame or almond, while Pitta individuals may benefit from cooling oils such as coconut or sunflower, and Kapha individuals may benefit from stimulating oils such as mustard or eucalyptus.

Facial Steam (Swedana)

Swedana is an Ayurvedic steam therapy that involves the use of herbs and spices. Facial steam (Mukha Swedana) is a popular Ayurvedic beauty ritual that involves steaming the face with a mixture of herbs such as neem, tulsi, and rose petals. Facial steam helps to open up the pores, promote circulation, and detoxify the skin. It also helps to balance the doshas and enhance the complexion. The type of herbs used for facial steam may vary based on the individual's dosha.

Herbal Face Pack (Mukha Lepa)

Mukha Lepa is an Ayurvedic herbal face pack that is made from natural ingredients such as turmeric, sandalwood, neem, and rose petals. The face pack is applied to the face and left on for a few minutes before being washed off. Mukha Lepa helps to detoxify the skin, remove impurities, and nourish the skin. It also helps to balance the doshas and enhance the complexion. The type of herbal face pack used may vary based on the individual's dosha.

Herbal Hair Treatment (Shiro Abhyanga)

Shiro Abhyanga is an Ayurvedic hair treatment that involves the use of warm herbal oils to massage the scalp and hair. The treatment helps to nourish the hair follicles, promote healthy hair growth, and reduce stress. The type of oil used for the hair treatment may vary based on the individual's dosha. For example, Vata individuals may benefit from warming oils such as sesame or almond, while Pitta individuals may benefit from cooling oils such as coconut or sunflower, and Kapha individuals may benefit from stimulating oils such as mustard or eucalyptus.

Herbal Bath (Snanam)

Snanam is an Ayurvedic herbal bath that involves the use of herbs and spices. The bath water is infused with herbs such as neem, tulsi, and rose petals. Snanam helps to detoxify the skin, reduce stress, and promote relaxation. It also helps to balance the doshas and enhance the complexion. The type of herbs used for the herbal bath may vary based on the individual's dosha.

Ayurvedic Diet

According to Ayurveda, diet plays a significant role in maintaining overall health and beauty. Ayurvedic diet recommendations are based on the individual's dosha. For example, Vata individuals may benefit from warm, nourishing foods such as soups and stews, Pitta individuals

Ayurvedic Massage and Bodywork

Ayurvedic Massage and Bodywork are an essential part of Ayurvedic healing practices, used for thousands of years to promote physical, mental, and emotional well-being. Ayurvedic Massage and Bodywork techniques are based on the principles of Ayurveda, which emphasizes the importance of maintaining a balance between the body, mind, and spirit for optimal health.

Ayurvedic Massage and Bodywork are known as Abhyanga in Sanskrit. Abhyanga is a form of massage that uses herbal oils and other natural ingredients to help balance the body's energy, improve circulation, stimulate the lymphatic system, and promote relaxation. Abhyanga is a full-body massage that includes the head, face, hands, and feet.

The Ayurvedic philosophy teaches that every person is unique and has a distinct body constitution, or Dosha, which influences their physical, mental, and emotional characteristics. Therefore, Ayurvedic Massage and Bodywork techniques are tailored to the individual's specific Dosha to help bring them into balance.

1. There are three primary Doshas in Ayurveda: Vata, Pitta, and Kapha. Each Dosha has unique characteristics, and Ayurvedic Massage and Bodywork techniques are tailored to balance the specific needs of each Dosha.

Vata Dosha is associated with movement and creativity. Vata types tend to be thin, light, and have dry skin. Ayurvedic Massage and Bodywork techniques for Vata types focus on nourishing the body and increasing circulation, using warm and grounding oils like sesame or almond oil.

Pitta Dosha is associated with transformation and digestion. Pitta types tend to have oily skin and a medium build. Ayurvedic Massage and Bodywork techniques for Pitta types focus on reducing inflammation, using cooling and calming oils like coconut or sunflower oil.

Kapha Dosha is associated with structure and stability. Kapha types tend to have a larger build and soft, oily skin. Ayurvedic Massage and Bodywork techniques for Kapha types focus on stimulating the body and reducing stagnation, using warm and invigorating oils like mustard or eucalyptus oil.

In addition to Abhyanga, there are several other Ayurvedic Massage and Bodywork techniques, including Shirodhara, Pinda Sweda, and Udvartana.

Shirodhara is a type of Ayurvedic therapy that involves pouring warm herbal oil over the forehead in a continuous stream. This technique is known for its ability to calm the mind, reduce stress and anxiety, and promote deep relaxation.

Pinda Sweda is a type of Ayurvedic massage that involves the application of warm, herb-infused poultices to the body. This technique helps to stimulate circulation, reduce inflammation, and relieve pain.

Udvartana is a type of Ayurvedic massage that involves the application of herbal powders to the body. This technique helps to stimulate circulation, remove toxins from the body, and reduce excess fat and cellulite.

In addition to promoting physical health, Ayurvedic Massage and Bodywork are also used to promote emotional and spiritual well-being. Ayurvedic practitioners believe that physical and emotional health are closely interconnected, and that massage and bodywork can help to release emotional blockages and promote a sense of inner peace.

Ayurvedic Massage and Bodywork can also be used in conjunction with other Ayurvedic practices, such as yoga, meditation, and herbal remedies, to promote overall health and well-being. By incorporating Ayurvedic Massage and Bodywork into your daily routine, you can help to bring your body, mind, and spirit into balance, promoting optimal health and well-being.

The role of massage in Ayurveda

Ayurveda, the ancient system of medicine from India, recognizes the benefits of massage as a way to balance the body and mind. Massage is considered an important tool in Ayurveda for promoting health and wellness, and is commonly used as part of Ayurvedic treatments and therapies.

According to Ayurveda, the body is made up of three doshas, or energies, which are responsible for different functions in the body. These doshas are Vata, Pitta, and Kapha, and each dosha is associated with different qualities and characteristics.

Massage is believed to help balance the doshas by increasing circulation, promoting relaxation, and stimulating the body's natural healing processes. Ayurvedic massage techniques focus on specific areas of the body, such as the feet, hands, head, and face, and use oils and herbs to help restore balance and harmony to the body and mind.

In Ayurveda, massage is considered to be an important part of a daily self-care routine, and is often used as a way to promote relaxation and reduce stress. It is believed that regular massage can help improve sleep quality, boost the immune system, and promote overall wellness.

Ayurvedic massage is often performed using warm herbal oils, which are chosen based on the individual's dosha type and any specific health concerns. The oils are selected for their therapeutic properties and are believed to help balance the doshas and support the body's natural healing processes.

One popular Ayurvedic massage technique is Abhyanga, which involves a full-body massage using warm herbal oils. During an Abhyanga massage, the therapist will use long, sweeping strokes to massage the body, focusing on areas where tension and stress are most commonly held.

Another Ayurvedic massage technique is Shirodhara, which involves the pouring of warm oil over the forehead and scalp. This technique is believed to promote relaxation and balance the doshas, and is often used as part of a larger Ayurvedic treatment plan.

Ayurvedic massage can also include techniques such as Marma therapy, which involves applying pressure to specific points on the body to promote healing and balance, and Pinda Sweda, which involves the use of warm herbal compresses to massage the body and promote relaxation.

In addition to promoting relaxation and reducing stress, Ayurvedic massage is also believed to help improve circulation, boost the immune system, and promote healthy skin. The oils used in Ayurvedic massage are often chosen for their skin-nourishing properties, and are believed to help promote healthy, radiant skin.

Ayurvedic massage techniques

Ayurveda, the traditional Indian system of medicine, considers massage to be an important part of maintaining good health. Ayurvedic massage, also known as Abhyanga, involves the use of warm herbal oils that are applied to the body in a rhythmic and gentle manner to promote relaxation, improve circulation, and detoxify the body. Ayurvedic massage techniques are designed to balance the three doshas, which are the three fundamental energies that govern the body and mind according to Ayurvedic principles.

Ayurvedic massage is believed to have a wide range of benefits for the body and mind. It is thought to help reduce stress, ease muscle tension, and promote deep relaxation. The warm herbal oils used in Ayurvedic massage are also believed to nourish and rejuvenate the skin, improve circulation, and support the immune system. In addition to these physical benefits, Ayurvedic massage is believed to have a calming effect on the mind, promoting mental clarity and emotional balance.

One of the key principles of Ayurvedic massage is the use of warm herbal oils. These oils are typically infused with a variety of herbs and spices that are selected according to the individual's dosha type. For example, sesame oil is commonly used in Ayurvedic massage for individuals with a Vata constitution, as it is believed to be warming and grounding. Coconut oil, on the other hand, is often used for individuals with a Pitta constitution, as it is cooling and soothing.

Ayurvedic massage techniques vary depending on the individual's dosha type and the specific needs of the person. However, there are some general techniques that are commonly used in Ayurvedic massage. These include:

Effleurage - This technique involves long, sweeping strokes that are used to warm up the muscles and prepare them for deeper massage. Effleurage is typically performed using light to moderate pressure.

Petrissage - This technique involves kneading and squeezing the muscles to release tension and improve circulation. Petrissage is often performed using deeper pressure than effleurage.

Friction - This technique involves rubbing the muscles in a circular motion to stimulate blood flow and improve muscle tone. Friction is typically performed using moderate to deep pressure.

Tapotement - This technique involves tapping or drumming on the muscles to release tension and stimulate circulation. Tapotement is often performed using light to moderate pressure.

In addition to these techniques, Ayurvedic massage may also involve the use of acupressure points, which are specific points on the body that are believed to correspond to different organs and systems in the body. By applying pressure to these points, the massage therapist can help to release tension and promote healing throughout the body.

Ayurvedic massage is typically performed in a warm and quiet environment, with the individual lying on a comfortable massage table. The massage therapist will apply warm herbal oils to the body and use a combination of massage techniques to promote relaxation and balance the doshas. The massage may also include the use of steam, hot towels, or other Ayurvedic treatments to enhance the overall experience.

Benefits of Ayurvedic bodywork

Ayurvedic bodywork, also known as Ayurvedic massage or Abhyanga, is an ancient healing technique that originated in India. It is a holistic approach to health and wellness, incorporating massage, herbal remedies, and dietary and lifestyle changes. Ayurvedic bodywork is based on the belief that the body, mind, and spirit are interconnected and that balance in these areas is essential for good health. Below we will explore the benefits of Ayurvedic bodywork.

One of the primary benefits of Ayurvedic bodywork is its ability to promote relaxation and reduce stress. The massage techniques used in Ayurvedic bodywork are gentle and rhythmic, which can help to calm the mind and reduce anxiety. This type of massage also promotes the release of endorphins, which are natural painkillers that help to reduce stress and promote a sense of well-being.

Another benefit of Ayurvedic bodywork is its ability to improve circulation. The massage techniques used in this practice help to increase blood flow and oxygen to the body's tissues, which can improve the function of organs and systems throughout the body. Improved circulation can also help to reduce inflammation, which is a common cause of pain and disease in the body.

Ayurvedic bodywork is also believed to help with detoxification. The massage techniques used in this practice help to stimulate the lymphatic system, which is responsible for removing toxins and waste from the body. This can help to improve immune function and reduce the risk of illness and disease.

In addition to these physical benefits, Ayurvedic bodywork is also believed to have psychological benefits. The gentle, rhythmic massage techniques used in this practice can help to calm the mind and promote a sense of inner peace. This can be especially beneficial for individuals who suffer from anxiety or depression.

Ayurvedic bodywork is also believed to help improve the health and appearance of the skin. The massage techniques used in this practice help to increase circulation to the skin, which can help to promote cell regeneration and reduce the appearance of fine lines and wrinkles. Ayurvedic oils and herbal remedies are also used during the massage to nourish and hydrate the skin, leaving it soft and supple.

The use of herbal remedies is an integral part of Ayurvedic bodywork. These remedies are tailored to the individual's specific needs based on their dosha, or body type. For example, individuals with a Vata dosha may benefit from warm sesame oil, while individuals with a Pitta dosha may benefit from coconut oil. Herbal remedies may also be used to address specific health concerns, such as joint pain, digestive issues, or insomnia.

Ayurvedic bodywork is a gentle and holistic approach to health and wellness that offers numerous benefits for both the body and mind. This practice promotes relaxation, improves circulation, promotes detoxification, and helps to improve the health and appearance of the skin. The use of herbal remedies tailored to the individual's dosha is also an important aspect of Ayurvedic bodywork, providing targeted support for specific health concerns. Whether you are looking to reduce stress, improve your overall health, or simply relax and unwind, Ayurvedic bodywork is a powerful tool for achieving your wellness goals.

Ayurvedic Aromatherapy

Ayurveda, the ancient Indian system of medicine, is a holistic approach to healing and maintaining health that encompasses many modalities. One such modality is aromatherapy, which involves the use of essential oils to promote physical, mental, and emotional well-being. In Ayurvedic aromatherapy, essential oils are chosen and used based on their properties and their effects on the doshas, the three biological humors that govern the body and mind.

Essential oils are highly concentrated plant extracts that are obtained through steam distillation, cold pressing, or solvent extraction. They are used for a variety of purposes, including aromatherapy, massage, and skincare. In Ayurveda, essential oils are believed to work on a subtle level to balance the doshas and promote overall health and well-being.

Ayurvedic aromatherapy uses a variety of essential oils, each with its own unique properties and benefits. Some of the most commonly used oils include:

1. Lavender: Known for its calming and relaxing properties, lavender is often used to soothe the mind and promote restful sleep. It is also believed to have a balancing effect on all three doshas.

2. Peppermint: Known for its cooling and invigorating properties, peppermint is often used to alleviate headaches and digestive issues. It is believed to have a balancing effect on the pitta dosha.

3. Eucalyptus: Known for its respiratory and immune-boosting properties, eucalyptus is often used to alleviate coughs and colds. It is believed to have a balancing effect on the kapha dosha.

4. Rose: Known for its uplifting and heart-opening properties, rose is often used to promote feelings of love, compassion, and gratitude. It is believed to have a balancing effect on the vata dosha.

5. Sandalwood: Known for its grounding and centering properties, sandalwood is often used to calm the mind and promote feelings of inner peace. It is believed to have a balancing effect on all three doshas.

Ayurvedic aromatherapy uses essential oils in a variety of ways, including inhalation, massage, and baths. Inhalation involves using a diffuser or inhaling the scent directly from the bottle. Massage involves diluting the essential oil in a carrier oil, such as sesame or coconut oil, and using it to massage the body. Baths involve adding a few drops of essential oil to a warm bath and soaking in the water.

Ayurvedic aromatherapy is believed to have many benefits for the body and mind. Some of these benefits include:

6. Balancing the doshas: Essential oils are believed to have a balancing effect on the doshas, helping to bring them back into balance and promote overall health and well-being.

7. Alleviating physical symptoms: Essential oils are often used to alleviate physical symptoms, such as headaches, digestive issues, and respiratory problems.

8. Promoting emotional well-being: Essential oils are believed to have a powerful effect on the emotions, helping to promote feelings of calm, relaxation, and joy.

9. Enhancing spiritual awareness: Essential oils are believed to have a subtle effect on the mind, helping to enhance spiritual awareness and promote a deeper connection to the divine.

In order to use Ayurvedic aromatherapy effectively, it is important to choose the right oils and use them in the right way. This often involves working with a qualified Ayurvedic practitioner who can help you choose the right oils and develop a personalized aromatherapy practice based on your individual needs and constitution.

The use of essential oils in Ayurveda

Ayurveda, the ancient Indian system of healing, considers the use of essential oils and aromatherapy as a crucial component in achieving overall health and wellness. The use of essential oils, known as aromatherapy, is based on the principle of using natural plant extracts to enhance physical, emotional, and spiritual well-being.

The use of essential oils in Ayurveda is grounded in the belief that the sense of smell can profoundly affect the mind and body. Essential oils are concentrated plant extracts that are obtained through steam distillation, cold pressing, or solvent extraction. They are highly potent and contain the natural aroma and healing properties of the plant from which they are derived.

In Ayurveda, essential oils are used for a variety of purposes, including improving digestion, reducing stress and anxiety, promoting restful sleep, and treating skin and hair issues. Each essential oil has unique properties and benefits, making it important to understand the properties of each oil before use.

One of the main principles of Ayurveda is the concept of the three doshas - vata, pitta, and kapha. Each dosha has its unique characteristics and can be balanced using essential oils. For example, vata individuals benefit from warming, grounding oils such as cinnamon, ginger, and frankincense, while pitta individuals benefit from cooling and soothing oils such as peppermint, lavender, and rose. Kapha individuals benefit from stimulating and invigorating oils such as eucalyptus, lemon, and grapefruit.

In Ayurvedic aromatherapy, essential oils are used in a variety of ways, including inhalation, massage, and baths. Inhalation involves using a diffuser or adding a few drops of essential oil to hot water and inhaling the steam. Massaging the body with essential oils is another common practice in Ayurveda, as it helps to calm the mind and soothe the body. Bathing with essential oils can also be a relaxing and rejuvenating experience.

Ayurveda emphasizes the importance of using high-quality, pure essential oils to achieve the best results. It is important to avoid synthetic fragrances and choose oils that are organic and ethically sourced. Essential oils should also be diluted with a carrier oil, such as coconut or almond oil, before use to prevent skin irritation.

Ayurvedic practitioners often create customized blends of essential oils based on an individual's dosha and specific health concerns. These blends can be used in a variety of ways, such as in massage oils, bath salts, and diffusers.

The use of essential oils in Ayurveda is considered safe when used appropriately. However, it is important to consult with an Ayurvedic practitioner before using essential oils, especially if you have a pre-existing health condition or are pregnant or breastfeeding.

Dosha-specific essential oils

Ayurveda, the ancient Indian system of medicine, recognizes that each person is unique and has a unique constitution or Prakriti. The constitution is made up of three Doshas, which are Vata, Pitta, and Kapha, and these determine one's physical, mental, and emotional characteristics. Each Dosha has its unique traits and is affected by external factors such as the environment, diet, and lifestyle. Ayurveda has a holistic approach to health and wellness and emphasizes balancing the Doshas to achieve optimal health. Essential oils are one of the natural remedies that Ayurveda recommends for balancing the Doshas. Here, we will discuss Dosha-specific essential oils and their benefits.

Vata Dosha: Vata is associated with the elements of air and space and is responsible for movement in the body. People with a Vata constitution tend to be creative, energetic, and restless. They may experience dry skin, constipation, and anxiety when the Dosha is out of balance. Ayurveda recommends the use of warming, grounding, and calming essential oils for balancing Vata. Essential oils that are beneficial for Vata Dosha include:

1. Sandalwood oil: Sandalwood oil has a grounding and calming effect on the body and mind. It is beneficial for reducing anxiety and promoting relaxation.

2. Ginger oil: Ginger oil has a warming effect and is beneficial for improving digestion and reducing bloating and gas.

3. Lavender oil: Lavender oil is a calming and soothing oil that is beneficial for reducing anxiety, promoting relaxation, and improving sleep quality.

4. Frankincense oil: Frankincense oil has a calming effect on the nervous system and is beneficial for reducing anxiety and promoting relaxation.

Pitta Dosha: Pitta is associated with the elements of fire and water and is responsible for digestion and metabolism. People with a Pitta constitution tend to be intelligent, ambitious, and competitive. They may experience skin rashes, inflammation, and digestive issues when the Dosha is out of balance. Ayurveda recommends the use of cooling, calming, and soothing essential oils for balancing Pitta. Essential oils that are beneficial for Pitta Dosha include:

5. Rose oil: Rose oil has a cooling effect on the body and is beneficial for reducing inflammation and skin irritation.

6. Peppermint oil: Peppermint oil has a cooling and refreshing effect on the body and is beneficial for improving digestion and reducing digestive issues such as bloating and gas.

7. Fennel oil: Fennel oil has a cooling effect on the body and is beneficial for reducing inflammation and digestive issues.

8. Jasmine oil: Jasmine oil has a cooling and calming effect on the body and mind and is beneficial for reducing anxiety and promoting relaxation.

Kapha Dosha: Kapha is associated with the elements of earth and water and is responsible for structure and stability in the body. People with a Kapha constitution tend to be calm, nurturing, and grounded. They may experience sluggish digestion, weight gain, and congestion when the Dosha is out of balance. Ayurveda recommends the use of warming, stimulating, and invigorating essential oils for balancing Kapha. Essential oils that are beneficial for Kapha Dosha include:

9. Eucalyptus oil: Eucalyptus oil has a stimulating effect on the body and is beneficial for reducing congestion and improving respiratory function.

10. Cinnamon oil: Cinnamon oil has a warming effect on the body and is beneficial for improving digestion and reducing bloating and gas.

11. Rosemary oil: Rosemary oil has a warming and stimulating effect on the body and is beneficial for improving circulation and reducing stiffness.

12. Lemon oil: Lemon oil has a stimulating effect on the body

Ayurvedic aromatherapy techniques and applications

Ayurvedic aromatherapy is the use of essential oils extracted from plants and herbs for therapeutic purposes. Aromatherapy has been used for thousands of years in Ayurvedic medicine to treat a variety of physical and emotional conditions. Essential oils are highly concentrated plant extracts that are believed to have a wide range of therapeutic properties.

The use of essential oils in Ayurvedic aromatherapy is based on the concept of the doshas, which are the three fundamental energies that govern the body and mind. According to Ayurveda, each person has a unique combination of the three doshas – Vata, Pitta, and Kapha – that determines their physical and mental characteristics, as well as their susceptibility to diseases.

Essential oils can help balance the doshas and promote physical and emotional well-being by affecting the five elements (earth, water, fire, air, and ether) that make up the body and mind. Each dosha is associated with specific elements, and certain essential oils can be used to balance each dosha.

Vata dosha is associated with the elements of air and ether and is responsible for movement, creativity, and flexibility. When out of balance, it can lead to anxiety, insomnia, and digestive problems. Essential oils that can help balance Vata dosha include ginger, cinnamon, patchouli, and sandalwood.

Pitta dosha is associated with the elements of fire and water and is responsible for metabolism, digestion, and transformation. When out of balance, it can lead to anger, inflammation, and skin problems. Essential oils that can help balance Pitta dosha include rose, lavender, peppermint, and fennel.

Kapha dosha is associated with the elements of earth and water and is responsible for stability, nourishment, and growth. When out of balance, it can lead to lethargy, congestion, and weight gain. Essential oils that can help balance Kapha dosha include eucalyptus, lemon, basil, and frankincense.

There are many ways to use essential oils in Ayurvedic aromatherapy. One of the most popular methods is through inhalation, which can be done by adding a few drops of essential oil to a diffuser or inhaling the aroma directly from the bottle. Essential oils can also be added to massage oils, bathwater, or skincare products to promote relaxation and balance.

Another popular Ayurvedic aromatherapy technique is called nasya, which involves the application of essential oils to the nasal passages. This technique is believed to help cleanse the sinuses, improve respiratory function, and balance the doshas.

In addition to inhalation and nasya, essential oils can also be used in Ayurvedic aromatherapy through topical application. Diluted essential oils can be applied to the skin during massage or added to skincare products to promote healthy skin and balance the doshas.

Ayurvedic aromatherapy is a natural and effective way to promote physical and emotional well-being. By using essential oils to balance the doshas, Ayurvedic aromatherapy can help improve digestion, reduce stress, and promote healthy skin and hair. Whether you are looking to improve your physical health or enhance your emotional well-being, Ayurvedic aromatherapy can be a valuable tool in your wellness arsenal.

Ayurveda and Mental Health

Ayurveda, a traditional system of medicine, recognizes the mind and body as an interconnected whole. In Ayurveda, mental health is not separate from physical health. It views the mind as an organ that needs proper care and attention, just like any other organ in the body. Mental health issues can have a profound effect on a person's overall well-being, which is why Ayurveda places significant importance on maintaining a healthy mind.

The three doshas, Vata, Pitta, and Kapha, play a crucial role in determining a person's mental health. Each dosha has a unique influence on the mind and can lead to various mental health imbalances. The following is a breakdown of the impact each dosha has on mental health:

1. Vata: Vata governs movement in the body and mind. It is responsible for creativity, enthusiasm, and excitement. However, when Vata is out of balance, it can lead to anxiety, fear, and restlessness.

2. Pitta: Pitta governs digestion and transformation in the body and mind. It is responsible for mental clarity, intelligence, and focus. However, when Pitta is out of balance, it can lead to anger, frustration, and irritability.

3. Kapha: Kapha governs stability and structure in the body and mind. It is responsible for emotional stability, calmness, and compassion. However, when Kapha is out of balance, it can lead to depression, attachment, and lethargy.

Ayurveda recognizes that mental health is a multi-dimensional issue that requires a holistic approach. A combination of dietary changes, lifestyle modifications, herbs, and practices can help restore balance and promote optimal mental health.

4. Dietary Changes: Ayurveda recommends eating a healthy, balanced diet that is appropriate for your dosha. A diet that is specific to your dosha can help promote mental balance and stability. Ayurveda recommends avoiding processed foods, refined sugar, and caffeine, as they can all lead to imbalances in the mind.

5. Lifestyle Modifications: Ayurveda emphasizes the importance of maintaining a healthy lifestyle to promote optimal mental health. This includes getting adequate sleep, engaging in regular physical activity, and managing stress. Daily practices such as meditation, yoga, and pranayama can help promote mental clarity and balance.

6. Herbs: Ayurveda has a vast array of herbs that can help promote optimal mental health. Ashwagandha, Brahmi, and Shankhpushpi are all examples of herbs that can help promote mental clarity and stability. These herbs can be taken in various forms, including capsules, teas, and powders.

7. Practices: Ayurveda has several practices that can help promote mental balance and stability. Abhyanga, or self-massage, is one such practice. This practice involves massaging the body with warm oil, which can help promote relaxation and calmness. Another practice is Shirodhara, which involves pouring warm oil over the forehead. This practice can help promote mental clarity and balance.

The Ayurvedic approach to mental health

Ayurveda, the ancient system of healing, recognizes the inseparable connection between the mind and the body. Ayurveda recognizes that mental and emotional wellbeing is crucial for overall health and that imbalances in the mind can contribute to physical ailments. In Ayurveda, the mind is seen as an extension of the body and is treated as such. This approach to mental health is unique and provides a holistic understanding of the mind-body connection. Below we will explore the Ayurvedic approach to mental health.

1. Ayurveda recognizes that the mind has three gunas or qualities: sattva, rajas, and tamas. These gunas are present in all aspects of life, including food, emotions, and thoughts. Sattva is the quality of purity, clarity, and harmony, while rajas is the quality of movement, change, and activity, and tamas is the quality of darkness, inertia, and negativity. The Ayurvedic approach to mental health focuses on achieving balance and harmony among these gunas.

One of the primary ways Ayurveda addresses mental health is through the concept of Dinacharya, or daily routine. A consistent daily routine can help to establish balance and stability in the mind and body. Dinacharya includes practices such as waking up and going to bed at the same time each day, practicing meditation or yoga, eating at regular times, and avoiding excessive stimulation, such as technology, before bed.

Another important Ayurvedic practice for mental health is the use of herbs and natural remedies. Ayurveda uses herbs such as ashwagandha, brahmi, and shankhapushpi to promote mental clarity and balance. These herbs are known for their calming and grounding effects on the mind, helping to alleviate stress, anxiety, and depression.

Ayurveda also emphasizes the importance of diet and nutrition in maintaining mental health. A diet that is balanced and nourishing for the body and mind is essential for mental wellbeing. Ayurvedic dietary guidelines include eating fresh, seasonal, and whole foods, avoiding processed and artificial foods, and eating mindfully and with intention.

In addition to these practices, Ayurveda also uses various therapies and treatments to address mental health issues. One such therapy is Shirodhara, a treatment that involves pouring a continuous stream of warm oil onto the forehead. This therapy is known for its calming and soothing effects on the mind and has been shown to be effective in treating anxiety, stress, and insomnia.

Ayurveda also recognizes the importance of emotional wellbeing in mental health. Ayurvedic practitioners believe that emotional imbalances can contribute to physical ailments and that emotional wellbeing is essential for overall health. Practices such as journaling, self-reflection, and connecting with nature can help to promote emotional balance and wellbeing.

In Ayurveda, the mind and body are seen as interconnected, and both must be in balance for optimal health. The Ayurvedic approach to mental health emphasizes the importance of daily routine, herbal remedies, nutrition, therapies, and emotional wellbeing in maintaining mental and emotional balance. By addressing the root causes of mental imbalances and promoting overall health and wellbeing, Ayurveda offers a unique and holistic approach to mental health that is both effective and sustainable.

Ayurvedic therapies for anxiety, depression, and stress

Ayurveda is an ancient Indian system of medicine that takes a holistic approach to health and wellness. It recognizes that mental health is an essential component of overall well-being and offers a range of therapies for managing anxiety, depression, and stress. These therapies include dietary changes, herbal remedies, lifestyle modifications, yoga, meditation, and other mind-body practices.

Anxiety, depression, and stress are widespread mental health issues that can significantly impact a person's quality of life. Ayurveda views mental health problems as imbalances in the doshas, or the body's natural energy systems. These imbalances can result from various factors, including poor diet, inadequate sleep, lack of exercise, and environmental stressors. Ayurvedic therapies aim to restore balance to the doshas and promote optimal mental health.

One of the most effective Ayurvedic therapies for anxiety, depression, and stress is dietary changes. The Ayurvedic diet emphasizes the consumption of whole foods that are fresh, organic, and seasonal. It also recognizes that each person's dietary needs may vary depending on their dosha type. For instance, individuals with a vata dosha may benefit from warm, nourishing foods, while those with a pitta dosha may benefit from cooling, calming foods. Ayurvedic practitioners may also recommend certain spices and herbs, such as turmeric and ashwagandha, which have been shown to have mood-enhancing properties.

Herbal remedies are another essential component of Ayurvedic therapies for mental health. Ayurvedic herbs have been used for thousands of years to support emotional well-being and improve overall health. Ashwagandha is one of the most commonly used Ayurvedic herbs for anxiety and depression. It has been shown to reduce stress and anxiety levels and improve overall mood. Brahmi is another herb that is frequently used to support mental health. It is known for its calming effects on the nervous system and has been shown to improve cognitive function and reduce anxiety and depression symptoms.

Lifestyle modifications are also critical in Ayurvedic therapies for mental health. Ayurvedic practitioners may recommend incorporating regular exercise into a person's daily routine, such as yoga or walking. Yoga is particularly beneficial for anxiety, depression, and stress, as it combines physical postures with breathwork and meditation. Regular yoga practice has been shown to reduce stress levels, improve mood, and enhance overall well-being. Ayurvedic practitioners may also recommend mindfulness practices, such as meditation and deep breathing exercises, to help manage symptoms of anxiety and depression.

Other Ayurvedic therapies for anxiety, depression, and stress include massage, acupuncture, and aromatherapy. Massage therapy can help promote relaxation, reduce tension, and improve overall mood. Acupuncture has been shown to reduce anxiety symptoms and improve overall well-being. Aromatherapy involves the use of essential oils to promote relaxation and reduce stress. Lavender and chamomile are two essential oils that are commonly used for anxiety and depression.

Supporting emotional well-being with Ayurveda

Ayurveda, the ancient Indian system of medicine, is a holistic approach to health and wellness that emphasizes the interconnectedness of the mind, body, and spirit. In Ayurveda, emotional well-being is considered an integral component of overall health, and there are a number of techniques and therapies that can be used to support emotional balance.

One of the key principles of Ayurveda is that each individual has a unique constitution, or dosha, which influences their physical, mental, and emotional tendencies. Understanding your dosha can help you to identify which therapies and techniques will be most effective for you.

One of the most effective ways to support emotional well-being in Ayurveda is through the use of herbs and other natural remedies. There are a number of herbs that are traditionally used in Ayurveda to support emotional balance, such as ashwagandha, brahmi, and shatavari. These herbs can be taken in various forms, such as capsules, teas, or tinctures, and can help to promote relaxation, calmness, and clarity of mind.

Another important aspect of emotional well-being in Ayurveda is the use of yoga and meditation. These practices can help to quiet the mind, reduce stress and anxiety, and promote feelings of inner peace and balance. In particular, restorative and gentle yoga poses, such as child's pose and forward folds, can be especially helpful for calming the mind and reducing anxiety.

In addition to yoga and meditation, there are a number of other Ayurvedic therapies that can be used to support emotional well-being. One of these is abhyanga, or Ayurvedic oil massage. This therapeutic massage uses warm herbal oils to help relax the muscles, soothe the nervous system, and promote a sense of calmness and well-being.

Another Ayurvedic therapy that is often used to support emotional balance is shirodhara, a traditional Ayurvedic treatment in which warm oil is poured over the forehead in a continuous stream. This treatment is deeply relaxing and can help to calm the mind and promote a sense of inner peace and tranquility.

Ayurveda also places great emphasis on diet and nutrition as a means of supporting emotional well-being. A diet that is rich in fresh, whole foods and balanced in accordance with your dosha can help to promote feelings of well-being and vitality. Foods that are considered particularly nourishing for the mind and emotions include fresh fruits and vegetables, whole grains, legumes, and nuts and seeds.

Finally, Ayurveda recognizes the importance of rest and relaxation in supporting emotional balance. Getting enough sleep, taking time for self-care, and cultivating healthy relationships and social connections are all important components of a balanced and healthy lifestyle.

Ayurveda for Women's Health

Ayurveda is an ancient holistic system of medicine that originated in India. Its philosophy revolves around the belief that the body, mind, and spirit are interconnected, and that the key to optimal health is balancing these elements. Ayurveda has long recognized the unique health needs of women and offers a range of strategies to support women's health and well-being.

One of the foundational principles of Ayurveda is the concept of the doshas, or the three vital energies that are believed to govern all physical and mental functions. The three doshas are vata, pitta, and kapha, and each dosha is associated with certain qualities and characteristics. Women, like all individuals, have a unique balance of doshas, and understanding this balance is key to supporting their health.

Ayurveda recognizes that women's health needs change throughout their lives, from menstruation to menopause and beyond. For example, during menstruation, women are believed to have a higher level of vata energy, which can lead to symptoms such as anxiety, fatigue, and insomnia. Ayurvedic strategies for balancing vata during this time might include eating warm, grounding foods, practicing gentle yoga, and getting adequate rest.

During menopause, women experience a decline in estrogen levels, which can lead to symptoms such as hot flashes, mood changes, and insomnia. Ayurvedic approaches to menopause focus on supporting the body's natural hormone production and helping to balance the doshas. For example, eating a balanced diet that includes phytoestrogen-rich foods, such as soy and flaxseeds, can help support hormone balance. Ayurvedic herbs such as ashwagandha and shatavari may also be helpful.

In addition to dietary and herbal interventions, Ayurveda offers a range of therapies and practices to support women's health. Abhyanga, or Ayurvedic oil massage, is a popular therapy that can help to balance the doshas and promote relaxation. Another popular therapy is shirodhara, which involves pouring a stream of warm oil over the forehead to calm the mind and balance the doshas.

Ayurveda also recognizes the importance of self-care practices for women's health. This includes developing a daily routine that supports overall well-being. A typical Ayurvedic routine might include waking up early, practicing yoga or meditation, eating a healthy breakfast, and taking time for self-care practices such as dry brushing or oil pulling.

In terms of dietary recommendations, Ayurveda emphasizes eating whole, fresh foods that are appropriate for an individual's dosha. For example, individuals with a vata-dominant constitution are encouraged to eat warm, grounding foods such as soups and stews, while those with a pitta-dominant constitution may benefit from cooling, hydrating foods such as salads and fruits.

Ayurveda also recognizes the importance of digestive health for overall well-being. Women are particularly prone to digestive issues such as bloating, constipation, and irritable bowel syndrome. Ayurvedic strategies for supporting digestive health include eating slowly and mindfully, avoiding cold drinks with meals, and incorporating digestive herbs such as ginger and fennel into the diet.

Finally, Ayurveda recognizes the importance of emotional well-being for overall health. Women may face a range of emotional challenges, from stress and anxiety to depression and grief. Ayurveda offers a range of practices to support emotional balance, including mindfulness meditation, journaling, and practices that promote self-awareness and self-acceptance.

Ayurvedic remedies for menstrual issues

Ayurveda, the ancient Indian system of medicine, offers a unique perspective on women's health, including menstrual issues. According to Ayurveda, a woman's menstrual cycle is a reflection of her overall health and well-being. Therefore, Ayurvedic remedies for menstrual issues focus on restoring balance to the body and promoting optimal health.

One of the most common menstrual issues is dysmenorrhea, or painful periods. Ayurveda attributes this to an imbalance in the body's vata dosha, which governs movement and circulation. To alleviate painful periods, Ayurveda recommends focusing on nourishing and grounding practices that support the body's ability to relax.

One of the most effective Ayurvedic remedies for menstrual pain is a warm oil massage, also known as Abhyanga. This involves using warm oil, such as sesame or coconut oil, to massage the lower abdomen and lower back. The warmth of the oil helps to improve circulation and reduce inflammation, while the massage itself can help to relax the muscles and promote a sense of calm.

Another Ayurvedic remedy for menstrual pain is the use of herbs and spices. Ginger is an excellent option, as it has anti-inflammatory properties that can help to reduce pain and discomfort. Drinking ginger tea or adding fresh ginger to meals can be helpful in reducing menstrual pain.

Fennel is another Ayurvedic herb that is commonly used for menstrual issues. Fennel seeds have a soothing effect on the digestive system and can help to relieve bloating and gas, which are common symptoms of premenstrual syndrome (PMS). Fennel tea is a simple and effective way to incorporate this herb into your routine.

In addition to herbal remedies, Ayurveda also emphasizes the importance of a balanced diet and lifestyle for optimal menstrual health. Eating a diet that is rich in whole foods and low in processed foods and sugar can help to support the body's natural detoxification processes and reduce inflammation.

Yoga and other gentle forms of exercise can also be beneficial for menstrual health. Practices such as restorative yoga and gentle stretching can help to improve circulation and promote relaxation, which can reduce menstrual pain and discomfort.

Ayurveda also recognizes the importance of emotional well-being in women's menstrual health. Stress and anxiety can have a significant impact on the menstrual cycle, and therefore Ayurveda emphasizes the importance of stress-reduction practices such as meditation and deep breathing.

In addition to menstrual pain, Ayurveda offers remedies for other common menstrual issues such as irregular periods, heavy bleeding, and PMS. Irregular periods are often a sign of an imbalance in the body's doshas, and Ayurveda offers a range of remedies to help restore balance. These include herbal remedies, such as ashoka, shatavari, and triphala, as well as lifestyle recommendations such as getting enough rest and reducing stress.

Heavy bleeding during menstruation is another common issue that can be addressed with Ayurvedic remedies. Ayurveda recommends incorporating foods that are rich in iron and other nutrients, such as leafy greens and beets, to support blood health. Herbs such as manjistha and turmeric can also be helpful in reducing inflammation and promoting healthy blood flow.

PMS is a collection of symptoms that can occur in the days leading up to menstruation, including bloating, mood swings, and fatigue. Ayurveda offers a range of remedies to help alleviate these symptoms, including dietary changes, herbal remedies, and stress-reduction practices such as meditation and yoga.

Supporting fertility and pregnancy with Ayurveda

Ayurveda, the ancient Indian system of medicine, has a long history of providing guidance and support for women's health, including fertility and pregnancy. According to Ayurveda, the health of the mother is crucial for the health of the child, and the child's constitution is determined by the balance of the mother's doshas (vata, pitta, and kapha) during pregnancy. Therefore, Ayurveda emphasizes the importance of balancing the doshas and maintaining overall health before and during pregnancy.

Ayurvedic Remedies for Fertility

Ayurveda offers various remedies for improving fertility and increasing the chances of conception. These remedies are based on the understanding that fertility is influenced by the balance of the doshas and the health of the reproductive tissues (shukra dhatu) in both men and women.

For women, Ayurvedic remedies for fertility often involve herbs and supplements that nourish the reproductive tissues and balance the hormones. Ashwagandha, shatavari, and gokshura are some of the commonly used herbs for promoting fertility in women. These herbs are believed to support the production of healthy eggs, regulate menstrual cycles, and improve the overall health of the reproductive system.

In addition to herbs, Ayurveda also emphasizes the importance of lifestyle changes and dietary modifications for improving fertility. This includes practices such as regular exercise, stress management, and a healthy diet that is rich in nutrients and antioxidants.

For men, Ayurvedic remedies for fertility focus on improving the quality and quantity of semen. Herbs such as ashwagandha, gokshura, and shatavari are also commonly used to promote healthy sperm production and improve sperm motility. In addition to herbs, Ayurveda also recommends a healthy diet, regular exercise, and stress management for improving male fertility.

Ayurvedic Support During Pregnancy

Ayurveda offers a comprehensive approach to supporting women's health during pregnancy. This approach involves a combination of diet, lifestyle, and herbal remedies that help to maintain balance and support the health of both the mother and the developing fetus.

One of the key aspects of Ayurvedic support during pregnancy is the use of herbal tonics and supplements that help to nourish the mother and support the growth and development of the fetus. Herbs such as shatavari, ashwagandha, and brahmi are commonly used during pregnancy to support the health of the mother and promote healthy fetal development.

Ayurveda also emphasizes the importance of maintaining a healthy diet during pregnancy. This includes eating a balanced and nourishing diet that is rich in nutrients such as protein, iron, and calcium. Ayurvedic practitioners may also recommend specific foods and spices that are believed to support the health of the mother and the developing fetus.

In addition to diet and herbal remedies, Ayurveda also emphasizes the importance of lifestyle modifications during pregnancy. This includes practices such as meditation, yoga, and regular exercise, which can help to reduce stress and promote relaxation.

Ayurvedic Remedies for Common Pregnancy Symptoms

Ayurveda offers various remedies for common pregnancy symptoms such as morning sickness, fatigue, and back pain. These remedies are generally safe and effective for pregnant women and are believed to help maintain balance and support overall health during pregnancy.

For example, ginger tea is a commonly recommended remedy for morning sickness in Ayurveda. Ginger is believed to help calm the stomach and reduce nausea and vomiting. Similarly, the use of massage and warm compresses can help to reduce back pain and improve circulation during pregnancy.

Ayurvedic care for postpartum and menopause

1. Ayurveda, the ancient Indian system of medicine, offers a comprehensive approach to women's health, from supporting menstrual health to managing menopause. The practice emphasizes a holistic approach to health and wellness, with a focus on balancing the body's natural energies, or doshas. Here we explore how Ayurveda can support women's health during two important stages of life: postpartum and menopause.

Postpartum Care in Ayurveda

Ayurveda offers a unique approach to postpartum care, known as the "confinement period." This period typically lasts for 42 days following delivery, during which new mothers are encouraged to rest, eat nourishing foods, and avoid strenuous activity. The aim of this period is to support the body in its recovery and to establish a healthy foundation for breastfeeding and caring for the newborn.

During the confinement period, Ayurveda recommends a diet rich in nutrient-dense foods, such as ghee, sesame oil, and soups made with root vegetables and spices. These foods are believed to nourish the body and promote healthy digestion. Additionally, Ayurvedic practitioners may recommend herbal supplements, such as shatavari and ashwagandha, to support hormonal balance and promote milk production.

In terms of self-care, Ayurveda recommends gentle oil massage, known as abhyanga, to support relaxation and promote healthy circulation. New mothers may also benefit from hot herbal baths, known as sitz baths, to promote healing and reduce inflammation. These practices can be particularly beneficial for women who have experienced a difficult delivery or who are struggling with postpartum depression or anxiety.

Managing Menopause with Ayurveda

Menopause is a natural and normal transition in a woman's life, but it can be accompanied by uncomfortable symptoms such as hot flashes, mood swings, and insomnia. Ayurveda offers a unique approach to managing menopause that focuses on supporting the body's natural balance.

According to Ayurveda, menopause represents a shift in the body's natural balance of the three doshas, with an increase in the vata dosha and a decrease in the kapha dosha. As a result, Ayurvedic practitioners may recommend lifestyle and dietary changes to support these changes in the body.

Dietary recommendations may include incorporating warming and grounding foods, such as cooked vegetables, whole grains, and healthy fats, into the diet. Additionally, Ayurvedic practitioners may recommend herbal supplements, such as ashwagandha and shatavari, to support hormonal balance and promote relaxation.

In terms of self-care, Ayurveda recommends incorporating gentle exercise, such as yoga and walking, into the daily routine to promote healthy circulation and balance the body's natural energies. Additionally, women may benefit from self-massage with warm sesame oil to support relaxation and promote healthy skin.

Ayurveda for Digestive Health

Ayurveda, the ancient Indian system of medicine, places great emphasis on digestive health. In Ayurveda, it is believed that proper digestion is the key to overall health and well-being. The digestive system is responsible for processing food and eliminating waste, and when it is functioning properly, the body can absorb essential nutrients and eliminate toxins effectively. However, when the digestive system is imbalanced, it can lead to a host of health issues, such as indigestion, constipation, and other digestive disorders. Ayurveda offers a range of remedies and practices to promote healthy digestion and support digestive health.

Ayurvedic Principles of Digestion

According to Ayurveda, the digestive system is composed of the digestive fire, or agni, which is responsible for breaking down food and converting it into usable energy. There are thirteen types of agni in Ayurveda, and each one corresponds to a specific stage of digestion. When the digestive fire is balanced, it allows for the efficient digestion of food, absorption of nutrients, and elimination of waste. However, when the digestive fire is weak or imbalanced, it can lead to digestive issues such as bloating, gas, and constipation.

Ayurvedic Remedies for Digestive Health

Ayurveda offers a range of remedies and practices to support healthy digestion. One of the most commonly used remedies is the use of spices in cooking. Spices such as ginger, cumin, coriander, and fennel are used to stimulate the digestive fire and promote healthy digestion. These spices can be added to meals or taken in the form of teas or supplements.

Another Ayurvedic remedy for digestive health is the use of herbal supplements. Herbs such as triphala, which is a blend of three fruits, are used to support healthy digestion and elimination. Triphala is believed to be effective in regulating bowel movements, reducing inflammation, and promoting the elimination of toxins.

In addition to spices and herbal supplements, Ayurveda also recommends specific dietary practices to support digestive health. It is recommended to eat meals at regular intervals and to avoid overeating. Meals should be consumed in a relaxed and peaceful environment, and it is important to avoid consuming cold or raw foods, as they can weaken the digestive fire.

Ayurvedic Practices for Digestive Health

Ayurveda also offers a range of practices to promote healthy digestion. One of the most commonly used practices is the practice of yoga. Yoga poses such as twists and forward bends are believed to stimulate the digestive organs and promote healthy digestion. In addition to yoga, Ayurveda also recommends the practice of pranayama, or breathing exercises, to support digestive health.

Another Ayurvedic practice for digestive health is the practice of self-massage, or abhyanga. This involves massaging the abdomen with warm oil in a clockwise direction, which is believed to stimulate the digestive fire and promote healthy digestion. Additionally, Ayurveda recommends the practice of mindfulness and relaxation techniques, such as meditation, to reduce stress and promote healthy digestion.

The Ayurvedic approach to digestion

Ayurveda, the ancient Indian system of medicine, has a holistic approach to health and wellness that emphasizes the importance of proper digestion. According to Ayurvedic philosophy, digestion is not just a physical process but also a mental and emotional one that is essential for overall health and well-being. Below we will explore the Ayurvedic approach to digestion and how it can help improve our overall health.

Ayurveda recognizes that digestion is the foundation of good health. When our digestion is strong and healthy, we are better able to absorb nutrients from our food and eliminate waste products efficiently. Ayurveda also recognizes that every individual has a unique digestive system, and that the type of food we eat, as well as our lifestyle habits, can have a significant impact on our digestion.

In Ayurveda, digestion is divided into three stages, called agni, which are responsible for different aspects of the digestive process. Jatharagni is the digestive fire located in the stomach and small intestine, responsible for breaking down food into its constituent parts. Bhutagni is the digestive fire located in the liver, responsible for processing and metabolizing nutrients. Finally, dhatvagni is the digestive fire located in the tissues, responsible for assimilating nutrients into the body's cells and eliminating waste products.

According to Ayurveda, imbalances in the digestive system can lead to a variety of health problems. These imbalances can be caused by a variety of factors, including stress, poor diet, lack of exercise, and environmental toxins. When the digestive system is not functioning properly, it can lead to a buildup of toxins in the body, which can cause a range of health problems, including fatigue, weight gain, and digestive disorders like bloating, constipation, and diarrhea.

1. One of the key principles of Ayurveda is that food is medicine. Ayurveda recognizes that different foods have different effects on the body and that choosing the right foods for your body type can help support healthy digestion. Ayurveda classifies foods into six different tastes: sweet, sour, salty, bitter, pungent, and astringent. Each of these tastes has different effects on the body, and Ayurvedic practitioners use this knowledge to create individualized meal plans for their clients.

In addition to choosing the right foods, Ayurveda also emphasizes the importance of eating in a relaxed and mindful manner. Eating when we are stressed or on-the-go can impair digestion and lead to a range of health problems. Ayurvedic practitioners recommend taking time to sit down and eat a meal in a calm and peaceful environment, free from distractions.

Ayurveda also recognizes the importance of regular exercise for maintaining healthy digestion. Exercise helps stimulate the digestive system and improves the body's ability to eliminate waste products. Ayurvedic practitioners recommend incorporating a variety of exercises into your daily routine, including yoga, walking, and strength training.

In addition to diet and exercise, Ayurveda also emphasizes the importance of managing stress for maintaining healthy digestion. Stress can have a significant impact on the digestive system, impairing its ability to function properly. Ayurvedic practitioners recommend incorporating stress-management techniques like meditation, breathing exercises, and relaxation techniques into your daily routine to help reduce stress levels and improve digestive health.

Finally, Ayurveda recognizes the importance of maintaining a healthy gut microbiome for healthy digestion. The gut microbiome is the community of bacteria that lives in our digestive tract, and it plays a critical role in digestion and overall health. Ayurvedic practitioners recommend incorporating fermented foods like yogurt, kefir, and sauerkraut into your diet to help support a healthy gut microbiome.

Ayurvedic remedies for common digestive issues

Ayurveda is an ancient Indian system of medicine that emphasizes the importance of balancing the body, mind, and spirit for optimal health. One of the key aspects of Ayurveda is the emphasis on digestive health, as the digestive system is seen as the foundation of overall well-being. Ayurvedic remedies for common digestive issues are aimed at restoring balance to the digestive system and promoting optimal digestion and absorption of nutrients. Below we will explore some of the most common digestive issues and the Ayurvedic remedies that can help to alleviate them.

One of the most common digestive issues is indigestion, which is characterized by discomfort or pain in the upper abdomen, bloating, and nausea. Ayurvedic remedies for indigestion include ginger, which can help to stimulate digestive enzymes and improve digestion. Ginger can be consumed in a variety of forms, including as a tea, added to meals, or taken as a supplement. Another effective Ayurvedic remedy for indigestion is fennel, which can help to reduce bloating and gas. Fennel can be consumed as a tea or added to meals as a spice.

Acid reflux is another common digestive issue that can be caused by the improper functioning of the lower esophageal sphincter. Ayurvedic remedies for acid reflux include licorice root, which can help to soothe the lining of the esophagus and reduce inflammation. Licorice root can be consumed as a tea or taken as a supplement. Another effective Ayurvedic remedy for acid reflux is aloe vera, which can help to soothe the digestive system and reduce inflammation. Aloe vera can be consumed as a juice or taken as a supplement.

Constipation is another common digestive issue that can be caused by a variety of factors, including a low-fiber diet, dehydration, and lack of physical activity. Ayurvedic remedies for constipation include triphala, which is a combination of three fruits that can help to promote bowel movements and improve digestive health. Triphala can be consumed as a powder or taken as a supplement. Another effective Ayurvedic remedy for constipation is psyllium husk, which can help to add bulk to the stool and promote regular bowel movements. Psyllium husk can be consumed as a powder or taken as a supplement.

Diarrhea is a common digestive issue that is characterized by loose, watery stools. Ayurvedic remedies for diarrhea include chamomile, which can help to soothe the digestive system and reduce inflammation. Chamomile can be consumed as a tea or taken as a supplement. Another effective Ayurvedic remedy for diarrhea is coconut water, which can help to rehydrate the body and provide electrolytes that are lost during diarrhea. Coconut water can be consumed as a beverage or added to meals as a base.

Supporting gut health with Ayurveda

Ayurveda, the ancient Indian system of medicine, places great emphasis on gut health. In Ayurveda, the digestive system is considered the foundation of health and well-being, with a healthy gut being essential for the proper functioning of the body and mind. Ayurvedic principles and practices can be used to support gut health and treat various digestive disorders. Let's take a closer look at how Ayurveda approaches gut health.

The Ayurvedic Approach to Digestion

In Ayurveda, digestion is seen as a process of transformation. Food is transformed into energy, bodily tissues, and waste products. Digestion is considered a complex process involving various bodily tissues, organs, and systems. Ayurveda recognizes that each individual has a unique digestive system and recommends personalized approaches to support gut health.

According to Ayurveda, there are three doshas or bio-energies that govern the body and mind - Vata, Pitta, and Kapha. Each of these doshas is associated with specific qualities and functions in the body, including digestion.

1. Vata Dosha and Digestion: Vata is responsible for the movement of food through the digestive system. When Vata is imbalanced, it can lead to irregular digestion, bloating, constipation, and gas.

2. Pitta Dosha and Digestion: Pitta is responsible for digestion and the transformation of food into energy. When Pitta is imbalanced, it can lead to acid reflux, heartburn, inflammation, and diarrhea.

3. Kapha Dosha and Digestion: Kapha is responsible for the lubrication and nourishment of the digestive system. When Kapha is imbalanced, it can lead to sluggish digestion, heaviness after meals, and weight gain.

Ayurvedic Remedies for Common Digestive Issues

Ayurveda recommends various remedies and practices to support gut health and treat common digestive issues. Here are some Ayurvedic remedies for digestive disorders:

4. Ginger: Ginger is a popular Ayurvedic remedy for digestive disorders. It is known for its ability to increase digestive fire, reduce inflammation, and relieve nausea. Ginger can be added to meals, tea, or taken as a supplement.

5. Triphala: Triphala is an Ayurvedic herbal formulation made from three fruits - amla, haritaki, and bibhitaki. It is known for its ability to improve digestion, relieve constipation, and detoxify the body.

6. Cumin: Cumin is another popular Ayurvedic spice that is used to support gut health. It is known for its ability to improve digestion, relieve bloating, and reduce inflammation. Cumin can be added to meals or taken as a supplement.

7. Probiotics: Probiotics are beneficial bacteria that are naturally present in the gut. They can help improve digestion, reduce inflammation, and support the immune system. Ayurveda recommends consuming probiotic-rich foods like yogurt, kefir, and fermented vegetables.

8. Fennel: Fennel is an Ayurvedic herb that is commonly used to support digestive health. It is known for its ability to relieve bloating, gas, and indigestion. Fennel can be added to meals, tea, or taken as a supplement.

Supporting Gut Health with Ayurveda

In addition to the above remedies, Ayurveda recommends various practices to support gut health. Here are some Ayurvedic practices for digestive health:

9. Eating Mindfully: Ayurveda recommends eating in a calm, relaxed environment and chewing food thoroughly. Mindful eating can help improve digestion, reduce stress, and prevent overeating.

10. Fasting: Fasting is an Ayurvedic practice that can help support gut health. It gives the digestive system a break, promotes detox

Ayurveda for Immunity

Ayurveda, the ancient Indian system of medicine, has a holistic approach towards health and well-being, which includes building a strong immune system. According to Ayurveda, immunity is referred to as "Ojas" and is considered to be a subtle essence that circulates throughout the body. Ojas is responsible for promoting physical and mental health, providing vitality, and fighting diseases. Thus, maintaining a strong immune system is crucial for overall health, and Ayurveda offers many techniques to boost immunity.

Ayurveda views the immune system as a complex web of interrelated processes that involve physical, mental, and emotional factors. In Ayurveda, immunity is related to the digestive system, and a healthy digestive system is believed to be the foundation of good health. According to Ayurveda, poor digestion can lead to the accumulation of toxins or "ama" in the body, which can impair the immune system. Therefore, Ayurveda emphasizes the importance of maintaining healthy digestion for optimal immune function.

One of the essential practices of Ayurveda for boosting immunity is to follow a balanced and nutritious diet. Ayurveda believes that food is not just a source of energy but also has medicinal properties. Thus, it is essential to eat a diet that is appropriate for one's body type or "dosha." Ayurveda recommends eating fresh, whole foods that are easy to digest and are in season. Foods that are rich in antioxidants, vitamins, and minerals, such as leafy greens, berries, nuts, and seeds, can also help to support the immune system.

In Ayurveda, herbs and spices are also used to support immunity. Some of the commonly used Ayurvedic herbs for boosting immunity include ashwagandha, turmeric, ginger, garlic, and tulsi. These herbs have immune-boosting properties and are also known for their anti-inflammatory and antioxidant effects. Ayurvedic practitioners may recommend taking these herbs in the form of supplements, teas, or incorporating them into meals.

Ayurveda also emphasizes the importance of lifestyle practices in promoting immunity. Regular exercise and physical activity are essential for maintaining good health and strengthening the immune system. Ayurveda recommends incorporating moderate exercise, such as yoga, walking, or swimming, into daily routines. Exercise helps to improve circulation, which can help to deliver oxygen and nutrients to the cells of the body and support immune function.

Another lifestyle practice recommended by Ayurveda for boosting immunity is stress management. Ayurveda recognizes that stress can have a detrimental effect on the immune system and overall health. Thus, Ayurveda recommends various techniques such as meditation, deep breathing, and yoga to manage stress and promote relaxation. These practices can help to reduce stress hormones such as cortisol and improve immune function.

In addition to these practices, Ayurveda also offers various therapies to support immunity. One such therapy is "Panchakarma," a detoxification process that involves a series of massages, herbal treatments, and other practices that help to remove toxins from the body. Panchakarma is believed to improve digestion, boost immunity, and promote overall health.

Another Ayurvedic therapy for boosting immunity is "Rasayana," which involves using specific herbs, oils, and other substances to promote longevity and rejuvenation. Rasayana therapies are believed to enhance the immune system, improve digestion, and promote overall well-being.

Ayurvedic principles for a strong immune system

Ayurveda, the ancient Indian system of medicine, emphasizes the importance of a strong immune system to maintain overall health and prevent diseases. According to Ayurveda, the immune system is the result of the balance between the three doshas - Vata, Pitta, and Kapha. When these doshas are in balance, the immune system functions optimally, but when they are imbalanced, the immune system weakens, making the body more susceptible to diseases.

Ayurveda recommends several principles to promote a strong immune system. One of the most important principles is to follow a healthy diet that is appropriate for your dosha. Ayurveda emphasizes the importance of eating fresh, whole foods that are rich in nutrients and free from toxins. Ayurvedic practitioners also recommend incorporating immune-boosting herbs and spices into your diet, such as turmeric, ginger, garlic, and holy basil.

In addition to following a healthy diet, Ayurveda recommends engaging in regular physical activity to support the immune system. Ayurvedic exercise, such as yoga, helps to balance the doshas and improve circulation, which can help to boost immunity. It's also important to get adequate rest and sleep to support the immune system. Ayurveda recommends getting seven to eight hours of sleep each night and establishing a regular sleep schedule.

Ayurveda also recommends several lifestyle practices to support a strong immune system. One of the most important is stress management. Stress weakens the immune system and makes the body more susceptible to diseases. Ayurvedic practitioners recommend engaging in practices such as meditation, pranayama, and mindfulness to reduce stress and support the immune system.

Ayurvedic practitioners also recommend practicing good hygiene habits to prevent the spread of diseases. Regularly washing your hands, avoiding touching your face, and covering your mouth when you cough or sneeze can all help to prevent the spread of germs.

Ayurveda also offers several specific remedies for boosting the immune system. One of the most popular remedies is the use of herbal supplements. Ayurvedic herbs, such as ashwagandha, guduchi, and amla, have been used for centuries to boost the immune system and improve overall health. These herbs can be taken in supplement form or incorporated into the diet.

Another popular Ayurvedic remedy for boosting immunity is the use of immune-boosting oils, such as sesame oil, ghee, and coconut oil. These oils can be used for cooking, as well as for self-massage, to promote circulation and boost immunity.

Ayurvedic practitioners may also recommend specific Ayurvedic treatments, such as panchakarma, to boost immunity. Panchakarma is a detoxification treatment that involves a series of therapeutic procedures to cleanse the body of toxins and restore balance to the doshas. This treatment is believed to improve overall health and boost the immune system.

Immune-boosting herbs and practices

Ayurveda, the ancient Indian system of medicine, emphasizes the importance of a strong immune system to maintain overall health and well-being. According to Ayurvedic principles, a strong immune system not only protects the body from infectious diseases but also promotes longevity and vitality.

There are several Ayurvedic practices and herbs that are known to boost the immune system. Below we will discuss some of these practices and herbs and their benefits in detail.

Ayurvedic Principles for a Strong Immune System

In Ayurveda, the immune system is closely linked to the concept of Ojas, which is considered to be the vital essence of the body. Ojas is responsible for maintaining overall health, immunity, and vitality. According to Ayurvedic principles, a strong immune system is the result of a balanced diet, regular exercise, healthy lifestyle practices, and a positive mental attitude.

Ayurveda also emphasizes the importance of a healthy digestive system for a strong immune system. In Ayurvedic terms, the digestive fire, or Agni, is responsible for breaking down the food we eat and converting it into energy. When Agni is strong, it helps to eliminate toxins from the body, which can otherwise weaken the immune system. Therefore, Ayurveda recommends eating a healthy, balanced diet that supports digestive health, such as whole grains, fresh fruits and vegetables, and lean protein.

Immune-Boosting Herbs and Practices in Ayurveda

Ashwagandha

Ashwagandha is an adaptogenic herb that is commonly used in Ayurveda to boost the immune system. It is believed to improve overall immunity by reducing stress, anxiety, and inflammation. Studies have shown that Ashwagandha can increase the number of white blood cells in the body, which are responsible for fighting off infections and diseases.

Turmeric

Turmeric is a popular spice in Ayurvedic medicine that is known for its anti-inflammatory and antioxidant properties. It contains a compound called curcumin, which is believed to boost the immune system by increasing the activity of immune cells in the body. Turmeric is commonly used in Ayurveda to treat respiratory infections, allergies, and digestive issues.

Tulsi

Tulsi, also known as Holy Basil, is an herb that is widely used in Ayurvedic medicine for its immune-boosting properties. It is believed to improve overall immunity by reducing stress, promoting mental clarity, and boosting the activity of immune cells in the body. Tulsi is commonly used in Ayurveda to treat respiratory infections, allergies, and skin disorders.

Yoga and Pranayama

Yoga and Pranayama, or breathing exercises, are both practices that are commonly used in Ayurveda to boost the immune system. Yoga is believed to improve overall health and well-being by reducing stress, improving circulation, and promoting relaxation. Pranayama, on the other hand, is a form of breathing exercise that is believed to improve lung function and boost the activity of immune cells in the body.

Oil Pulling

Oil pulling is an ancient Ayurvedic practice that involves swishing oil around in the mouth to improve oral health and boost the immune system. It is believed to improve overall immunity by removing toxins and harmful bacteria from the mouth, which can otherwise weaken the immune system.

Triphala

Triphala is an Ayurvedic herbal supplement that is commonly used to improve digestive health and boost the immune system. It contains three herbs, Amla, Haritaki, and Bibhitaki, that are known for their antioxidant and anti-inflammatory properties. Triphala is believed to improve overall immunity by supporting digestive health, which in turn strengthens the immune system.

Seasonal immunity support

Ayurveda, the ancient Indian system of medicine, emphasizes the importance of maintaining good health and preventing diseases through a balanced lifestyle and diet. One of the key aspects of Ayurvedic health is immunity support, which can help us stay healthy and fight off infections and illnesses. In Ayurveda, immunity is understood as the body's natural defense against disease-causing pathogens, and there are various ways to strengthen and support this defense.

One of the fundamental principles of Ayurveda is the concept of doshas, which are the three energies that govern the body's functions and determine our physical and mental characteristics. Each dosha, namely Vata, Pitta, and Kapha, has a unique set of qualities and tendencies that influence our health and wellbeing. Ayurveda recognizes that maintaining the balance of the doshas is crucial for a healthy immune system.

The first step in supporting our immunity according to Ayurveda is to eat a balanced and wholesome diet that nourishes our body and mind. The food we eat should be fresh, seasonal, and tailored to our dosha type. Ayurveda recommends including immune-boosting foods such as fresh fruits and vegetables, whole grains, nuts, seeds, and spices in our daily diet. Some of the best immune-boosting herbs and spices in Ayurveda include turmeric, ginger, garlic, cinnamon, and ashwagandha.

Another critical aspect of Ayurvedic immunity support is following a healthy daily routine that balances the doshas and promotes overall wellbeing. This includes waking up early in the morning, practicing yoga or meditation, and getting enough sleep at night. Ayurvedic practices such as oil pulling, tongue scraping, and nasal cleansing can also help remove toxins from the body and boost immunity.

Ayurveda also recognizes the importance of seasonal changes in our health and wellbeing. Each season has its unique qualities, and Ayurveda recommends adapting our diet and lifestyle accordingly to maintain a healthy immune system. For instance, during the winter season, it is essential to eat warm, nourishing foods and keep the body warm and protected from the cold. In contrast, during the summer season, we need to stay hydrated, eat cooling foods, and protect ourselves from the sun's heat.

Ayurveda offers many natural remedies and practices to support immunity and prevent diseases. One such practice is Ayurvedic herbal formulations, known as rasayanas, which are designed to nourish the body and strengthen immunity. Some popular Ayurvedic rasayanas include Chyawanprash, Amrit Kalash, and Triphala. These formulations contain a blend of herbs, spices, and other natural ingredients that have immune-boosting properties.

Ayurveda also recognizes the importance of regular exercise in maintaining good health and immunity. Exercise helps to strengthen the body and mind, improve digestion, and promote overall wellbeing. Ayurveda recommends practicing yoga, walking, or other moderate exercises that are appropriate for our body type and dosha.

Lastly, Ayurveda emphasizes the importance of managing stress and emotional wellbeing for maintaining good immunity. Stress and negative emotions can weaken the immune system and make us susceptible to diseases. Ayurveda recommends various practices such as meditation, mindfulness, and pranayama to manage stress and promote emotional wellbeing.

Ayurveda for Pain Management

Ayurveda, the ancient Indian science of healing, offers a comprehensive approach to pain management. Pain is a common symptom that affects millions of people worldwide, and Ayurveda provides a holistic and natural approach to treating pain without relying on pharmaceutical drugs. Ayurveda emphasizes the connection between the mind and the body, and its approach to pain management involves identifying the underlying causes of pain and addressing them through natural remedies and lifestyle changes.

According to Ayurveda, pain is caused by an imbalance of the doshas, or the three fundamental energies that govern all bodily functions. The three doshas are Vata, Pitta, and Kapha, and they represent the elements of air, fire, and earth, respectively. Each person has a unique constitution, or Prakriti, which is determined by the dominant dosha or combination of doshas. Imbalances in the doshas can cause pain and other health problems.

Ayurvedic pain management focuses on restoring balance to the doshas and promoting overall health and wellness. One of the primary approaches to pain management in Ayurveda is through diet and lifestyle changes. Ayurveda recommends a diet that is suitable for the individual's Prakriti, as well as incorporating spices and herbs that have anti-inflammatory and analgesic properties. Additionally, practicing regular exercise and maintaining good sleep hygiene can help balance the doshas and promote overall well-being.

Ayurveda also utilizes various natural remedies to relieve pain. One of the most popular remedies is the use of herbal oils and massage therapy. Ayurvedic massage, or Abhyanga, involves the application of warm oil to the body, followed by gentle massage. The warm oil helps to soothe the muscles and joints, while the massage helps to improve circulation and reduce pain. Ayurvedic herbs such as ginger, turmeric, and boswellia have also been used for centuries to alleviate pain and inflammation.

In addition to diet, lifestyle changes, and natural remedies, Ayurveda also emphasizes the importance of mental and emotional well-being in pain management. Stress and anxiety can exacerbate pain symptoms, and Ayurveda recognizes the mind-body connection in health and wellness. Ayurveda promotes practices such as meditation, yoga, and pranayama (breathing exercises) to help manage stress and improve mental and emotional health.

Ayurveda also recognizes that pain management is a personalized approach, and the remedies and treatments that work for one person may not work for another. Therefore, Ayurveda emphasizes the importance of individualized treatment plans that take into account a person's unique constitution and specific health concerns. Ayurvedic practitioners work with their patients to develop personalized treatment plans that address the root causes of pain and promote overall health and well-being.

Ayurvedic pain management has been used for centuries to alleviate various types of pain, including joint pain, back pain, headaches, and menstrual pain. Unlike pharmaceutical drugs, which can have negative side effects and may only provide temporary relief, Ayurvedic remedies and lifestyle changes focus on restoring balance to the doshas and promoting overall health and well-being. While Ayurvedic pain management may not work for everyone, it provides a safe and natural alternative to traditional pharmaceutical drugs and offers a comprehensive approach to pain management.

The Ayurvedic approach to pain relief

Ayurveda, the ancient Indian system of medicine, takes a holistic approach to health and wellness, and this includes the management of pain. In Ayurveda, pain is viewed as a result of an imbalance in the body, and the focus is on addressing the root cause of the imbalance rather than just masking the pain. This approach is different from that of modern medicine, which often relies on painkillers and other medications to manage pain.

According to Ayurveda, the body is composed of three doshas or energies - Vata, Pitta, and Kapha. Each dosha governs different functions in the body, and an imbalance in one or more of these doshas can lead to pain. For example, an excess of Vata can cause joint pain, while an excess of Pitta can cause inflammation and heat in the body, leading to pain. Similarly, an excess of Kapha can lead to a feeling of heaviness and sluggishness, which can also contribute to pain.

The Ayurvedic approach to pain relief involves balancing the doshas and promoting the body's natural healing mechanisms. This can be achieved through a combination of dietary and lifestyle changes, along with specific Ayurvedic treatments.

Diet plays a crucial role in Ayurvedic pain management. Eating a balanced diet that is tailored to an individual's dosha can help to prevent imbalances that can lead to pain. For example, those with a Vata imbalance may benefit from warm, nourishing foods such as soups and stews, while those with a Pitta imbalance may benefit from cooling foods such as cucumber and watermelon. Kapha types may benefit from a diet that is light and easy to digest, with plenty of herbs and spices to stimulate digestion.

Lifestyle changes can also be beneficial for managing pain in Ayurveda. Regular exercise is important for maintaining the health of the muscles and joints, but it is essential to choose the right type of exercise based on one's dosha. For example, those with a Vata imbalance may benefit from gentle exercise such as yoga, while those with a Pitta imbalance may benefit from more vigorous activities such as running or swimming. Kapha types may benefit from regular movement throughout the day to prevent stagnation and promote circulation.

Ayurvedic treatments such as massage, herbal remedies, and meditation can also be helpful for managing pain. Massage is particularly beneficial for those with Vata imbalances, as it helps to soothe the nervous system and promote relaxation. Herbal remedies such as turmeric, ginger, and ashwagandha can be used to reduce inflammation and promote healing in the body. Meditation and other relaxation techniques can also help to reduce stress and promote a sense of calm, which can be beneficial for managing pain.

In addition to these general principles, there are also specific Ayurvedic treatments for different types of pain. For example, oil massage can be particularly effective for managing joint pain, while steam therapy can be helpful for reducing stiffness and improving mobility. Ayurvedic treatments such as Shirodhara, a form of massage that involves pouring warm oil on the forehead, can also be helpful for reducing stress and promoting relaxation, which can in turn help to manage pain.

Ayurvedic therapies for pain management

Ayurveda, the ancient Indian system of medicine, has a holistic approach to pain management. In Ayurveda, pain is seen as an imbalance in the body's doshas (vata, pitta, and kapha), and the goal of treatment is to restore balance to the doshas and eliminate the underlying cause of the pain. Ayurvedic therapies for pain management are gentle, natural, and effective, and can be used in conjunction with modern medical treatments.

Ayurvedic therapies for pain management include:

1. Abhyanga Massage: Abhyanga is a type of Ayurvedic massage that involves the use of warm herbal oils to massage the body. Abhyanga massage helps to calm the mind, reduce stress, and improve circulation. It also helps to reduce pain and stiffness in the joints and muscles.

2. Panchakarma: Panchakarma is a detoxification treatment in Ayurveda. It involves a series of therapies that help to remove toxins from the body and restore balance to the doshas. Panchakarma can be particularly effective in treating chronic pain conditions such as arthritis, fibromyalgia, and back pain.

3. Yoga and Meditation: Yoga and meditation are essential components of Ayurvedic therapy. Yoga postures and breathing exercises help to improve flexibility, strength, and balance, and can reduce pain and inflammation in the body. Meditation can help to calm the mind and reduce stress, which can also help to alleviate pain.

4. Herbal Remedies: Ayurveda uses a variety of herbs and spices to treat pain. Turmeric, ginger, and ashwagandha are commonly used for their anti-inflammatory properties. Boswellia is used to reduce joint pain and inflammation. Guggulu is used to reduce pain and stiffness in the muscles.

5. Diet and Lifestyle Changes: Ayurveda emphasizes the importance of diet and lifestyle in managing pain. Eating a balanced diet that is rich in fruits, vegetables, whole grains, and lean protein can help to reduce inflammation in the body. Getting regular exercise, practicing stress-reducing techniques such as yoga and meditation, and getting enough sleep can also help to reduce pain and improve overall health.

Ayurvedic therapies for pain management are safe and gentle, and can be used by people of all ages. However, it is important to consult with a qualified Ayurvedic practitioner before starting any new treatment. Ayurvedic therapies are not a substitute for medical care, and should be used in conjunction with modern medical treatments.

Managing chronic pain with Ayurveda

Ayurveda, the ancient system of medicine, has a holistic approach to pain management, which focuses on restoring balance to the body, mind, and spirit. Chronic pain, which can be defined as pain that lasts for longer than three months, can be debilitating and negatively impact a person's quality of life. Ayurveda offers a range of therapies that can help manage chronic pain, including dietary and lifestyle modifications, herbal remedies, and specialized body treatments.

1. According to Ayurveda, pain is caused by an imbalance in the body's doshas, or energy forces. There are three doshas in Ayurveda: Vata, Pitta, and Kapha. Each dosha is associated with specific physical and emotional traits and imbalances can cause various health issues, including pain.

Vata dosha is responsible for movement and is associated with dryness, coldness, and roughness. When there is an imbalance in Vata, it can cause pain, stiffness, and numbness. Pitta dosha, on the other hand, is associated with heat, light, and transformation. When Pitta is imbalanced, it can cause inflammation and burning sensations, leading to pain. Kapha dosha is associated with stability, structure, and lubrication. When Kapha is imbalanced, it can cause dull, heavy, and achy pain.

To manage chronic pain, Ayurveda recommends identifying the root cause of the pain and addressing it through dietary and lifestyle modifications. For example, if Vata dosha is imbalanced and causing pain, it is recommended to avoid cold and dry foods and opt for warm, nourishing foods. Gentle exercise, such as yoga and walking, can also be beneficial in managing Vata-related pain.

Ayurvedic herbal remedies can also be helpful in managing chronic pain. Turmeric, ginger, and ashwagandha are known for their anti-inflammatory and analgesic properties and can be incorporated into the diet or taken as supplements. Ayurvedic oils, such as sesame or coconut oil, can be used for self-massage to help alleviate pain and stiffness.

In addition to dietary and herbal remedies, Ayurveda offers specialized body treatments, such as Panchakarma, to manage chronic pain. Panchakarma is a detoxification and rejuvenation treatment that involves a combination of herbal remedies, massage, and other therapies to balance the doshas and remove toxins from the body. Panchakarma can be effective in managing chronic pain caused by imbalances in the doshas.

Ayurveda also emphasizes the importance of managing stress and emotions, as chronic pain can be exacerbated by stress and emotional imbalances. Meditation, pranayama, and other relaxation techniques can be helpful in managing stress and promoting emotional well-being.

Ayurveda for Weight Management

Ayurveda, the ancient Indian system of medicine, has a holistic approach to weight management that focuses on balancing the body and mind. According to Ayurveda, each individual has a unique body constitution, or "prakriti," which determines their metabolic rate, digestion, and energy levels. Therefore, the approach to weight management in Ayurveda is personalized, taking into account one's body type, lifestyle, and eating habits.

One of the fundamental principles of Ayurveda for weight management is maintaining a balance of the three doshas - Vata, Pitta, and Kapha. Each dosha has a unique set of characteristics, and imbalances in any of these can lead to weight gain. Therefore, an Ayurvedic weight management plan focuses on correcting any imbalances and restoring the natural balance of the doshas.

In Ayurveda, weight gain is often associated with an imbalance of Kapha dosha. Kapha is responsible for stability, structure, and lubrication in the body. When Kapha is out of balance, it can lead to sluggish digestion, water retention, and accumulation of toxins in the body, leading to weight gain. Therefore, an Ayurvedic approach to weight management often involves reducing Kapha through diet, lifestyle changes, and specific herbs and supplements.

One of the key dietary recommendations for weight management in Ayurveda is to eat according to one's dosha. For example, those with a Kapha-predominant constitution should avoid heavy, oily, and sweet foods, and instead focus on light, dry, and spicy foods to balance the dosha. Similarly, those with a Vata or Pitta constitution have their specific dietary guidelines for weight management.

Another important aspect of Ayurvedic weight management is physical activity. According to Ayurveda, regular exercise helps balance the doshas and promotes digestion and metabolism. However, the type of exercise recommended may vary based on one's dosha. For example, those with a Vata constitution may benefit from gentle and calming exercises like yoga or tai chi, while those with a Pitta constitution may benefit from more intense and challenging exercises like running or weight lifting.

In addition to diet and exercise, Ayurveda also recommends several herbs and supplements for weight management. Some of the commonly used herbs in Ayurvedic weight management include Triphala, Guggulu, and Shilajit. These herbs help support digestion, metabolism, and detoxification in the body, helping to promote weight loss.

Ayurvedic weight management also emphasizes the importance of mindful eating and awareness of one's body. Ayurveda suggests eating in a calm and peaceful environment, free from distractions, and taking time to chew food properly to aid digestion. Practicing mindfulness and being aware of one's hunger and fullness cues can also help prevent overeating and promote healthy weight management.

Ayurvedic principles for maintaining a healthy weight

Ayurveda, the ancient Indian system of medicine, places great emphasis on maintaining a healthy weight for overall well-being. According to Ayurveda, being overweight or underweight can lead to imbalances in the body, which can manifest as various health problems. Below we will discuss the Ayurvedic principles for maintaining a healthy weight.

In Ayurveda, the concept of a healthy weight is not based solely on a person's body mass index (BMI). Instead, it takes into account an individual's constitution, or dosha, which is determined by the balance of the three doshas - vata, pitta, and kapha - in the body. Each dosha has a unique set of characteristics, and imbalances in the doshas can lead to weight gain or loss.

According to Ayurveda, excess weight is typically associated with the kapha dosha, which is characterized by heaviness, slow metabolism, and a tendency towards lethargy. People with a kapha-dominant constitution tend to gain weight easily and have difficulty losing it. On the other hand, a vata-dominant person may struggle with maintaining a healthy weight due to a fast metabolism and a tendency towards irregular eating patterns.

Ayurvedic principles for maintaining a healthy weight focus on balancing the doshas through diet, lifestyle, and herbal remedies. Here are some of the key principles:

1. Follow a dosha-specific diet: Ayurveda recommends following a diet that is tailored to your dosha to maintain a healthy weight. For example, a kapha-pacifying diet should include foods that are light, warm, and dry, such as spices, vegetables, and legumes. A vata-pacifying diet should include warm, nourishing foods, such as cooked grains, root vegetables, and healthy fats.

2. Practice mindful eating: Ayurveda emphasizes the importance of being present and fully engaged in the eating process. Mindful eating involves savoring each bite, chewing food thoroughly, and avoiding distractions such as television or phone screens. It also involves eating in a calm and peaceful environment, without rushing or multitasking.

3. Get regular exercise: Exercise is an important component of weight management in Ayurveda. However, the type and intensity of exercise should be tailored to the individual's dosha. For example, a kapha-dominant person may benefit from vigorous exercise that increases metabolism and circulation, while a vata-dominant person may need more gentle, grounding exercises such as yoga or walking.

4. Use herbal remedies: Ayurveda uses a variety of herbs and spices to support healthy weight management. For example, triphala, a combination of three fruits, is a common Ayurvedic remedy for weight loss. It is believed to improve digestion, reduce inflammation, and eliminate toxins from the body. Other herbs such as guggulu and ginger may also be used to support healthy weight management.

5. Maintain a regular routine: Ayurveda emphasizes the importance of maintaining a regular routine to balance the doshas and maintain a healthy weight. This includes going to bed and waking up at the same time each day, eating meals at regular times, and establishing a consistent exercise routine.

In addition to these Ayurvedic principles, it is important to seek the guidance of a qualified Ayurvedic practitioner for personalized recommendations. A practitioner can help identify imbalances in the doshas and develop a tailored plan for maintaining a healthy weight.

Dosha-specific weight management strategies

1. Ayurveda, the ancient Indian system of medicine, offers a personalized approach to weight management based on an individual's unique constitution or dosha. According to Ayurveda, there are three primary doshas: Vata, Pitta, and Kapha, each with its own unique characteristics and tendencies.

For those with a dominant Vata dosha, weight gain can be challenging as they tend to have a faster metabolism and may struggle to maintain weight. To manage weight, Vata-dominant individuals should focus on consuming warm, cooked foods that are grounding and nourishing. They should also aim to maintain a regular meal schedule and avoid skipping meals or fasting, which can aggravate Vata.

Individuals with a dominant Pitta dosha tend to have a more muscular build and can gain weight easily if they consume too many heavy, oily, or spicy foods. To maintain a healthy weight, Pitta-dominant individuals should focus on consuming cooling and hydrating foods, such as fresh fruits and vegetables. They should also avoid overeating and aim to eat smaller, more frequent meals throughout the day.

Kapha-dominant individuals tend to have a slower metabolism and can gain weight easily if they consume too many sweet, heavy, or oily foods. To manage weight, Kapha-dominant individuals should focus on consuming lighter, drier, and more spicy foods. They should also aim to maintain an active lifestyle and engage in regular exercise, as well as avoid excessive sleep or sedentary behavior.

Ayurveda also emphasizes the importance of proper digestion and elimination for maintaining a healthy weight. To improve digestion, individuals should eat in a calm and relaxed environment, avoid overeating, and consume foods that are easy to digest. To promote healthy elimination, individuals should consume plenty of water, engage in regular exercise, and maintain a daily routine that promotes regular bowel movements.

In addition to diet and lifestyle modifications, Ayurveda also offers various natural remedies and therapies to support weight management. Some common Ayurvedic remedies for weight management include drinking warm water with lemon juice and honey, consuming triphala powder or capsules, and taking ginger or cinnamon supplements.

Ayurvedic therapies for weight management may include herbal steam baths, massage therapy, and detoxification treatments. Herbal steam baths, known as swedana, are believed to help eliminate toxins from the body and promote weight loss. Massage therapy, or abhyanga, can help stimulate circulation and improve digestion, while detoxification treatments, such as panchakarma, can help remove deep-seated toxins and balance the doshas.

Ayurvedic remedies for weight loss

Ayurveda, the ancient Indian system of medicine, offers a holistic approach to weight loss. Rather than focusing on calorie counting and restrictive diets, Ayurveda considers the whole person and their unique constitution, or dosha, when creating a weight loss plan. Ayurvedic remedies for weight loss include dietary changes, herbal remedies, lifestyle modifications, and detoxification practices.

The three doshas, or mind-body types, in Ayurveda are Vata, Pitta, and Kapha. Each dosha has unique qualities and tendencies that can impact weight gain and loss.

Vata types tend to have a lean frame, fast metabolism, and variable appetite. However, when imbalanced, Vata can cause irregular digestion and weight loss resistance. To balance Vata and support healthy weight loss, Ayurveda recommends warming, nourishing foods, such as cooked grains, root vegetables, and healthy fats. Herbal remedies like ginger and fennel can help improve digestion and increase metabolism. Vata types may also benefit from a regular routine that includes regular meals, consistent exercise, and stress-reducing practices like yoga and meditation.

Pitta types are typically of medium build and have a strong appetite and digestion. However, when imbalanced, Pitta can lead to inflammation, acid reflux, and excess weight gain. To balance Pitta and support healthy weight loss, Ayurveda recommends cooling, hydrating foods, such as fresh fruits, vegetables, and whole grains. Herbal remedies like turmeric and aloe vera can help reduce inflammation and support digestion. Pitta types may also benefit from limiting spicy or acidic foods, getting regular exercise, and practicing stress management techniques.

Kapha types tend to have a larger frame, slow metabolism, and strong cravings. When imbalanced, Kapha can lead to weight gain, sluggish digestion, and water retention. To balance Kapha and support healthy weight loss, Ayurveda recommends light, spicy foods, such as steamed vegetables, lean protein, and warming spices like ginger and cinnamon. Herbal remedies like guggulu and triphala can help improve digestion and metabolism. Kapha types may also benefit from regular exercise, stimulating yoga practices like Sun Salutations, and incorporating more variety and excitement into their routine.

Ayurvedic remedies for weight loss also include lifestyle modifications that can support overall health and well-being. Getting enough sleep and managing stress levels are important factors in weight management, as chronic stress can lead to increased cortisol levels and weight gain. Regular exercise, such as yoga or walking, can improve circulation, metabolism, and digestion. Ayurvedic self-massage, or abhyanga, can also improve digestion and lymphatic flow, supporting weight loss and overall health.

Detoxification practices are also an important part of Ayurvedic weight loss. Ayurveda recommends seasonal detoxification, or panchakarma, to remove toxins from the body and reset the digestive system. This process involves a series of cleansing practices, including oil massage, herbal steam, and specialized dietary protocols.

In addition to these Ayurvedic remedies, it is important to seek the guidance of a qualified Ayurvedic practitioner when embarking on a weight loss journey. An Ayurvedic practitioner can help identify your unique dosha and create a customized plan that addresses your individual needs and goals. They can also provide ongoing support and guidance as you navigate the process of healthy weight loss.

Ayurveda for Aging Gracefully

Ayurveda is a holistic health system that originated in India thousands of years ago. Its primary goal is to help individuals achieve optimal health and well-being by focusing on the whole person - body, mind, and spirit. One important aspect of Ayurveda is its emphasis on aging gracefully. In Ayurveda, the aging process is seen as a natural and inevitable part of life, and there are a number of practices and remedies that can help individuals age gracefully and maintain good health as they grow older.

The Ayurvedic approach to aging gracefully is centered on the idea of balance. According to Ayurveda, aging is primarily caused by imbalances in the body and mind. These imbalances can be caused by a number of factors, including poor diet, lack of exercise, stress, and environmental toxins. To promote healthy aging, Ayurveda emphasizes the importance of balancing these factors through diet, lifestyle, and other natural remedies.

One key aspect of the Ayurvedic approach to aging gracefully is the concept of Rasayana. Rasayana is a Sanskrit term that means "rejuvenation" or "restoration." In Ayurveda, Rasayana refers to a specific set of practices and remedies that are designed to promote healthy aging and maintain good health in the elderly. These practices and remedies can include dietary changes, herbal remedies, massage, yoga, and meditation.

Diet is an important component of the Ayurvedic approach to aging gracefully. According to Ayurveda, a healthy diet should be based on the individual's dosha, or body type. Each dosha has its own specific dietary recommendations, but in general, a healthy Ayurvedic diet should be rich in fresh fruits and vegetables, whole grains, lean proteins, and healthy fats. It should also be low in processed foods, sugar, and artificial ingredients.

Herbal remedies are another important part of the Ayurvedic approach to aging gracefully. There are a number of Ayurvedic herbs that are believed to have anti-aging properties, including ashwagandha, guduchi, and amalaki. These herbs can be taken in the form of supplements or added to food as spices. In addition to these herbs, Ayurveda also emphasizes the importance of regular detoxification to rid the body of toxins and promote healthy aging.

Massage is another important component of the Ayurvedic approach to aging gracefully. Ayurvedic massage, known as Abhyanga, is a gentle form of massage that uses warm oils and gentle pressure to stimulate the body's natural healing processes. This type of massage can help to improve circulation, promote relaxation, and reduce stress.

Yoga and meditation are also important components of the Ayurvedic approach to aging gracefully. Yoga is a gentle form of exercise that can help to improve flexibility, balance, and strength. It can also help to reduce stress and improve overall well-being. Meditation, on the other hand, is a powerful tool for reducing stress, promoting relaxation, and improving mental clarity.

The Ayurvedic perspective on aging

1. Ayurveda, an ancient Indian system of medicine, views aging as a natural process that occurs throughout life. According to Ayurvedic principles, each individual is unique and possesses a unique combination of physical, mental, and emotional characteristics. These characteristics are known as doshas, which are composed of the five elements: ether, air, fire, water, and earth. As we age, our doshas change, which can lead to imbalances and health problems. Therefore, Ayurveda emphasizes the importance of maintaining a healthy balance of doshas throughout life to promote healthy aging.

2. Ayurveda identifies three doshas: Vata, Pitta, and Kapha. Vata is composed of air and ether and is associated with movement, Pitta is composed of fire and water and is associated with digestion and metabolism, and Kapha is composed of earth and water and is associated with stability and structure. Each dosha is associated with different physical, mental, and emotional characteristics, and imbalances in these doshas can lead to various health problems.

The Ayurvedic perspective on aging recognizes that each dosha has its own unique aging process. Vata is associated with dryness, stiffness, and thinning of tissues, leading to joint pain and osteoporosis. Pitta is associated with inflammation and heat, leading to skin aging and wrinkles. Kapha is associated with sluggishness and excess weight, leading to poor circulation and joint pain.

Ayurveda recommends several lifestyle practices to promote healthy aging, such as following a balanced diet, regular exercise, getting enough restful sleep, and practicing stress-management techniques. Ayurvedic practitioners may also recommend specific herbs and supplements to support healthy aging.

One of the key principles of Ayurvedic aging is maintaining a healthy digestive system. Ayurveda views the digestive system as the root of health and well-being, and therefore, emphasizes the importance of eating healthy, whole foods and supporting digestion with herbs and supplements. Ayurveda also recommends regular detoxification practices, such as fasting or cleansing diets, to remove toxins from the body and support overall health.

Another important aspect of Ayurvedic aging is the practice of self-care. Ayurveda recognizes the importance of taking care of oneself physically, mentally, and emotionally. This can include practicing yoga and meditation, receiving regular Ayurvedic massages or other body treatments, and engaging in activities that bring joy and fulfillment.

Ayurvedic practitioners may also recommend specific herbs and supplements to support healthy aging. Some of the most commonly used herbs in Ayurveda for aging include ashwagandha, guduchi, and shatavari. These herbs are believed to support healthy aging by promoting overall wellness and vitality.

Ayurvedic practices for longevity

Ayurveda, the ancient Indian system of medicine, offers a holistic approach to health and longevity. According to Ayurveda, the key to living a long and healthy life lies in achieving balance and harmony within oneself and with the environment. Ayurvedic practices for longevity are designed to promote physical, mental, and spiritual well-being, and to help individuals maintain a healthy and fulfilling life.

One of the fundamental principles of Ayurveda is the concept of doshas, which are the three fundamental energies that govern the body and mind. These doshas are Vata, Pitta, and Kapha, and they correspond to the elements of air, fire, and water, respectively. Each person has a unique combination of these doshas, which influences their physical and mental characteristics, as well as their susceptibility to disease.

To promote longevity, Ayurveda recommends that individuals maintain a balance of these doshas through diet, lifestyle, and other practices. For example, a Vata-predominant individual may benefit from warm, grounding foods, such as cooked vegetables and grains, and a regular routine that includes sufficient rest and relaxation. A Pitta-predominant individual, on the other hand, may benefit from cooling foods, such as fresh fruits and vegetables, and a daily exercise routine that promotes balance and calm. A Kapha-predominant individual may benefit from light, warming foods, such as spicy soups and stews, and regular movement and exercise to promote energy and vitality.

In addition to maintaining a balance of the doshas, Ayurveda emphasizes the importance of promoting healthy digestion and eliminating toxins from the body. Ayurvedic practices for digestion include eating in a calm and peaceful environment, chewing food thoroughly, and avoiding processed and refined foods. Ayurvedic detoxification practices include daily practices such as drinking warm lemon water in the morning, practicing yoga and meditation, and incorporating herbs such as triphala, ginger, and turmeric into the diet.

Ayurveda also recommends the use of rasayanas, which are rejuvenating substances that help to promote longevity and vitality. Rasayanas can be herbs, spices, or other natural substances that have been traditionally used in Ayurveda for their nourishing and rejuvenating properties. Popular rasayanas include ghee, ashwagandha, shatavari, and amalaki.

Another important aspect of Ayurvedic practices for longevity is maintaining a healthy and balanced mind. Ayurveda recognizes the connection between the mind and body, and emphasizes the importance of mental and emotional well-being in promoting overall health and longevity. Practices such as meditation, yoga, and pranayama can help to calm the mind and reduce stress, while positive affirmations and visualization techniques can help to promote a positive outlook and promote a sense of purpose and fulfillment in life.

Promoting cognitive health with Ayurveda

Ayurveda, the ancient Indian system of medicine, offers a holistic approach to maintaining optimal health, including cognitive health. The Ayurvedic approach emphasizes the importance of a healthy lifestyle and diet, regular exercise, and stress management. By following Ayurvedic principles, it is believed that one can achieve a balance between the mind, body, and spirit, leading to overall well-being.

1. The Ayurvedic approach to cognitive health begins with the recognition of the three doshas: Vata, Pitta, and Kapha. Each dosha represents a different combination of the five elements, and individuals are believed to have a dominant dosha, which affects their physical and mental characteristics. For cognitive health, it is important to balance the doshas to ensure that the mind is clear, focused, and alert.

One way to support cognitive health in Ayurveda is through the use of specific herbs and spices. For example, Brahmi (Bacopa monnieri) is a well-known herb in Ayurveda that is believed to improve cognitive function, memory, and learning. Ashwagandha (Withania somnifera) is another popular herb that is used to reduce stress and improve cognitive function. Turmeric (Curcuma longa) is a spice that is known for its anti-inflammatory properties and may also help support cognitive health.

Another important aspect of Ayurvedic cognitive health is the practice of yoga and meditation. These practices are believed to help calm the mind, reduce stress, and improve cognitive function. Yoga and meditation also help balance the doshas by increasing the flow of prana (life force energy) throughout the body.

Ayurvedic massage is another practice that may support cognitive health. Abhyanga, an Ayurvedic oil massage, is believed to help nourish the nervous system and promote relaxation. It is believed that regular Abhyanga massages can help reduce stress and anxiety, leading to improved cognitive function.

In addition to these practices, Ayurveda also emphasizes the importance of diet for cognitive health. It is recommended to consume fresh, whole foods that are rich in nutrients and antioxidants. Foods that are particularly beneficial for cognitive health include fruits and vegetables, nuts and seeds, whole grains, and healthy fats such as ghee and coconut oil.

Ayurveda also recommends avoiding processed foods, sugar, and caffeine, as these can negatively impact cognitive health. It is also important to eat in moderation and to avoid overeating, which can lead to digestive issues that can further affect cognitive function.

In Ayurveda, it is believed that cognitive health is linked to overall health and well-being. By following Ayurvedic principles, individuals can support cognitive health by promoting balance and harmony in the mind, body, and spirit. Through the use of herbs and spices, yoga and meditation, massage, and a healthy diet, one can support cognitive function and maintain optimal overall health.

Integrating Ayurveda into Modern Life

Ayurveda is an ancient Indian system of holistic medicine that has been practiced for thousands of years. The word Ayurveda is derived from two Sanskrit words: 'Ayur,' which means life, and 'Veda,' which means knowledge. Thus, Ayurveda translates to 'the science of life.' It is based on the belief that good health is a balance between mind, body, and spirit, and that any imbalance in these areas can lead to illness or disease. Ayurveda offers a comprehensive approach to health and wellness, and its principles can be integrated into modern life to promote overall well-being.

Ayurveda focuses on achieving and maintaining a balance of the three doshas, which are Vata, Pitta, and Kapha. Each person is believed to have a unique combination of these doshas, and when these are in balance, one experiences optimal health. Ayurveda also emphasizes the importance of a healthy digestive system, as digestion is believed to be the root of good health. Thus, Ayurvedic principles for integrating into modern life revolve around maintaining dosha balance and promoting healthy digestion.

One of the most important Ayurvedic principles for modern life is establishing a daily routine or 'dinacharya.' This includes practices such as waking up early, performing self-massage, practicing yoga or other physical exercise, and meditation. These practices help to balance the doshas and promote overall health and well-being. It is also important to establish a regular eating routine, as Ayurveda places great emphasis on the role of digestion in maintaining health. Eating at the same time each day and consuming warm, cooked foods can promote optimal digestion and balance the doshas.

Another important Ayurvedic principle is the use of herbs and spices to support health and wellness. Ayurveda has a rich tradition of using herbs and spices for medicinal purposes, and many of these can be easily incorporated into modern life. For example, ginger can aid digestion, turmeric can reduce inflammation, and ashwagandha can support the nervous system. Including these herbs and spices in daily meals can promote overall health and well-being.

Ayurveda also emphasizes the importance of mindful eating. This means taking time to eat slowly and savoring each bite, as well as being aware of the quality and quantity of food consumed. This practice can promote optimal digestion, prevent overeating, and help to maintain a healthy weight.

In addition to these practices, Ayurveda also offers a range of therapies and treatments for specific health issues. For example, Panchakarma is a traditional Ayurvedic detoxification and rejuvenation treatment that can help to cleanse the body of toxins and promote overall health. Shirodhara is a therapy that involves pouring warm oil over the forehead and can promote relaxation and reduce stress.

One of the challenges of integrating Ayurveda into modern life is the fast-paced and often stressful nature of modern living. Ayurveda offers a range of practices that can help to reduce stress and promote relaxation, such as meditation, yoga, and breathing exercises. These practices can be easily incorporated into daily life, even if only for a few minutes each day. Additionally, Ayurvedic massage and bodywork can help to reduce stress and promote relaxation, and can be received on a regular basis to promote overall health and well-being.

Combining Ayurveda with conventional medicine

Ayurveda, the traditional system of medicine from India, has been gaining popularity as a complementary approach to conventional medicine in recent years. The holistic approach of Ayurveda and its focus on prevention and balance aligns well with the principles of modern medicine, making it a valuable addition to healthcare. Below we will discuss the benefits of combining Ayurveda with conventional medicine and how it can be integrated into modern life.

Ayurveda focuses on the individual as a whole, taking into account not just the physical body but also the mind and spirit. This holistic approach can be beneficial in managing chronic conditions that may have a psychosomatic component, such as anxiety, depression, and stress. By addressing the root cause of the condition and working towards balancing the body and mind, Ayurvedic therapies can complement conventional treatment and enhance its effectiveness.

One of the primary benefits of integrating Ayurveda with conventional medicine is the personalized approach to treatment. Ayurveda recognizes that every individual is unique and requires a tailored approach to their healthcare. By taking into account an individual's constitution, current health status, and lifestyle, an Ayurvedic practitioner can design a treatment plan that is specific to the individual's needs. This approach can lead to better outcomes and a more personalized approach to healthcare.

Ayurveda also offers a range of natural therapies that can be used in conjunction with conventional treatments to promote healing and balance. These therapies include herbal remedies, massage, yoga, and meditation. These natural therapies can help to reduce the side effects of conventional treatments, such as chemotherapy, and improve overall quality of life.

Another benefit of integrating Ayurveda with conventional medicine is the emphasis on prevention. Ayurveda recognizes the importance of maintaining balance in the body and mind to prevent illness from occurring. By making lifestyle changes and incorporating Ayurvedic practices into daily life, individuals can work towards preventing chronic conditions from developing. This approach can be particularly beneficial for individuals with a family history of certain diseases or those with risk factors for chronic conditions such as diabetes or heart disease.

However, it is important to note that Ayurveda should not be used as a substitute for conventional medicine in emergency situations or for serious illnesses. In such cases, conventional medicine should always be the first line of treatment. Ayurveda can be used in conjunction with conventional medicine to promote healing and improve overall well-being.

To integrate Ayurveda into modern life, individuals can start by incorporating simple Ayurvedic practices into their daily routine. These practices include eating a balanced diet, practicing yoga and meditation, and getting adequate rest. Ayurvedic practitioners can also provide personalized recommendations based on an individual's constitution and health status.

Cultivating an Ayurvedic mindset

Cultivating an Ayurvedic mindset means adopting a holistic approach to health and wellness, emphasizing balance and harmony in all aspects of life. Ayurveda is an ancient Indian system of medicine and wellness that has gained popularity in recent years for its natural and personalized approach to health. Ayurvedic principles are based on the belief that everyone is unique, and therefore requires a personalized approach to health and wellness. Below we will explore the key principles of Ayurveda and how they can be applied to cultivate an Ayurvedic mindset for optimal health and well-being.

One of the fundamental principles of Ayurveda is that the mind and body are interconnected, and that one cannot be healthy without the other. In Ayurveda, the mind is seen as a powerful tool that can be used to cultivate good health and prevent illness. This is why cultivating an Ayurvedic mindset is so important. By focusing on the mind-body connection and taking a holistic approach to health, we can promote well-being and prevent disease.

Another important principle of Ayurveda is that everyone is unique and requires an individualized approach to health and wellness. This is because Ayurveda recognizes that everyone has a unique constitution, or dosha, that determines their physical, mental, and emotional characteristics. The three doshas are vata, pitta, and kapha, and each person has a unique combination of these doshas. By understanding your dosha, you can determine the best approach to diet, exercise, and lifestyle for optimal health and well-being.

Ayurveda also emphasizes the importance of balance and harmony in all aspects of life. This means finding a balance between work and rest, activity and relaxation, and social interaction and alone time. By finding balance in our daily lives, we can reduce stress and promote overall well-being.

In Ayurveda, diet and nutrition play a crucial role in maintaining health and preventing illness. Ayurvedic principles emphasize the importance of eating fresh, whole foods that are appropriate for your dosha. For example, those with a vata dosha are encouraged to eat warm, nourishing foods that are grounding and calming, while those with a pitta dosha are advised to eat cooling, refreshing foods that balance their fiery nature. Kapha doshas are encouraged to eat light, warming foods that promote digestion and metabolism. By eating according to our dosha, we can support our bodies and promote optimal health.

Ayurveda also recognizes the importance of physical activity in maintaining health and well-being. However, Ayurvedic principles emphasize that the type of exercise you do should be appropriate for your dosha. Those with a vata dosha may benefit from gentle, grounding exercises like yoga or tai chi, while those with a pitta dosha may enjoy more vigorous activities like running or weight lifting. Kapha doshas may benefit from more invigorating activities like dancing or martial arts. By finding the right type of exercise for your dosha, you can support your physical health and prevent illness.

In addition to diet and exercise, Ayurveda emphasizes the importance of self-care and relaxation in maintaining optimal health. This includes practices like meditation, massage, and aromatherapy, which can promote relaxation and reduce stress. By taking time for self-care, we can support our mental and emotional health and prevent illness.

While Ayurveda is a powerful system for promoting health and well-being, it is important to note that it should not be used as a replacement for conventional medicine. Instead, Ayurveda can be used in conjunction with conventional medicine to promote optimal health and prevent illness. By combining the principles of Ayurveda with modern medicine, we can take a holistic approach to health that considers the mind, body, and spirit.

Adapting Ayurveda to your lifestyle and needs

Ayurveda is an ancient system of medicine that has been practiced in India for thousands of years. It emphasizes the interconnectedness of the mind, body, and spirit and aims to restore balance and harmony to these aspects of our being. One of the unique aspects of Ayurveda is its focus on personalized treatment plans, tailored to the individual's unique constitution or dosha.

1. Adapting Ayurveda to your lifestyle and needs involves understanding your dosha and incorporating Ayurvedic principles into your daily routine. There are three primary doshas: Vata, Pitta, and Kapha. Each dosha is associated with specific physical and emotional traits, and understanding your dominant dosha can help you determine the types of foods, exercises, and self-care practices that will support your health and well-being.

To determine your dosha, an Ayurvedic practitioner will typically conduct a thorough assessment that includes questions about your diet, sleep habits, digestion, energy levels, and other aspects of your physical and emotional health. They may also observe your body type, skin, eyes, and tongue to get a sense of your unique constitution.

Once you know your dosha, you can begin to incorporate Ayurvedic practices into your daily routine. Here are some tips for adapting Ayurveda to your lifestyle and needs:

Eat for your dosha

Ayurveda places a strong emphasis on the role of food in maintaining health and well-being. Different doshas require different types of foods, so it's essential to eat for your dosha. For example, Vata types may benefit from warm, nourishing foods, while Pitta types may do better with cooling, soothing foods. Kapha types may benefit from light, energizing foods that help stimulate digestion.

Create a morning routine

A consistent morning routine can help set the tone for your day and support your overall health and well-being. Ayurveda recommends starting your day with a glass of warm water to stimulate digestion and eliminate toxins. You may also want to incorporate practices like oil pulling, tongue scraping, and gentle yoga or stretching.

Practice self-care

Self-care is an essential aspect of Ayurveda, and it can take many forms, depending on your dosha and unique needs. For Vata types, self-care may involve warm oil massages and meditation. Pitta types may benefit from cooling practices like swimming or spending time in nature. Kapha types may benefit from energizing practices like dancing or vigorous exercise.

Incorporate Ayurvedic herbs and supplements

Ayurvedic herbs and supplements can be a helpful way to support your overall health and well-being. For example, Ashwagandha is a powerful adaptogen that can help reduce stress and anxiety. Turmeric is a potent anti-inflammatory that can support joint health and digestion. Triphala is a combination of three herbs that can help support healthy digestion and elimination.

Prioritize rest and relaxation

Rest and relaxation are critical for maintaining good health, and Ayurveda emphasizes the importance of getting enough sleep and downtime. Aim to go to bed and wake up at the same time each day, and create a calming bedtime routine to help promote restful sleep. You may also want to incorporate practices like meditation, gentle yoga, or deep breathing into your daily routine to help reduce stress and promote relaxation.

Building an Ayurvedic Home

Ayurveda is an ancient Indian system of medicine that aims to balance the body, mind, and spirit to promote health and well-being. One way to incorporate Ayurveda into daily life is by creating an Ayurvedic home, which is a space that supports the body's natural rhythms and promotes optimal health. Below we will explore the principles of building an Ayurvedic home and how to incorporate them into daily life.

One of the main principles of an Ayurvedic home is to create a space that promotes relaxation and reduces stress. This can be achieved by designing a space that is clutter-free, well-lit, and airy. The use of natural materials, such as wood and stone, can also help create a calming environment. Soft lighting, candles, and incense can also be used to create a relaxing atmosphere.

Another important aspect of an Ayurvedic home is creating a space that supports healthy eating habits. The kitchen is the heart of the home and should be designed to promote healthy eating habits. This can be achieved by stocking the kitchen with fresh fruits and vegetables, whole grains, and healthy fats. Cooking with herbs and spices can also help promote good digestion and support overall health.

In Ayurveda, the bedroom is considered to be the most important room in the house as it is where the body repairs and rejuvenates itself. To create a bedroom that supports optimal health, it is important to create a space that is calm, quiet, and free of distractions. Soft lighting, comfortable bedding, and natural materials can all help promote restful sleep.

Another key principle of an Ayurvedic home is to create a space that promotes physical activity. Exercise is an important part of Ayurveda, and a home that promotes physical activity can help support overall health and well-being. This can be achieved by incorporating a home gym, yoga studio, or meditation space into the home.

In addition to physical activity, an Ayurvedic home should also promote mindfulness and meditation. This can be achieved by creating a space that is quiet and free of distractions, such as a meditation room or outdoor space. Incorporating natural elements, such as plants and water features, can also help promote a sense of calm and tranquility.

Finally, an Ayurvedic home should be designed to promote community and social connection. This can be achieved by creating spaces that encourage social interaction, such as a comfortable living room or outdoor patio. Creating a space for family meals and gatherings can also help promote a sense of community and connection.

Ayurvedic principles for a harmonious living space

Ayurveda is an ancient Indian science of healing that emphasizes the interconnectedness of the mind, body, and spirit. According to Ayurveda, creating a harmonious living space is essential for maintaining overall health and wellbeing. This article will explore some of the Ayurvedic principles for a harmonious living space and how they can be incorporated into your home.

The five elements of Ayurveda are earth, water, fire, air, and ether. These elements are believed to exist in everything, including the human body and the environment. To create a harmonious living space, Ayurveda recommends balancing these elements in your home.

One way to balance the elements in your home is through color. Each color is associated with a different element and has a specific effect on the mind and body. For example, earthy tones such as brown and green are associated with the earth element and can create a sense of grounding and stability. Blue and silver are associated with the water element and can create a sense of calmness and relaxation. Red and orange are associated with the fire element and can create a sense of energy and warmth. Yellow and white are associated with the air element and can create a sense of lightness and clarity. Finally, purple and black are associated with the ether element and can create a sense of space and openness.

Another way to balance the elements in your home is through the use of natural materials. Ayurveda recommends using natural materials such as wood, stone, and clay to create a sense of harmony and balance. These materials are believed to have a grounding effect and can help to connect you to the earth element.

Ayurveda also recommends creating a clutter-free living space. Clutter is believed to create a sense of chaos and can disrupt the flow of energy in your home. To create a clutter-free living space, Ayurveda recommends simplifying your belongings and keeping only the things that are essential. This can help to create a sense of calm and order in your home.

In addition to creating a clutter-free living space, Ayurveda also recommends incorporating plants into your home. Plants are believed to have a purifying effect on the air and can help to balance the elements in your home. Certain plants, such as lavender and jasmine, are also believed to have a calming effect on the mind and body.

Finally, Ayurveda recommends incorporating aromatherapy into your home. Certain essential oils are believed to have a balancing effect on the mind and body and can help to create a sense of harmony in your living space. For example, lavender oil is believed to have a calming effect, while peppermint oil is believed to have an energizing effect.

Using Vastu Shastra to create balance in your home

Using Vastu Shastra to Create Balance in Your Home

Vastu Shastra, a traditional Hindu system of architecture, is often described as the science of harmony between humans and the environment. It emphasizes the importance of creating a balanced living space that promotes health, happiness, and prosperity. Vastu Shastra is rooted in the principles of Ayurveda, the ancient Indian system of medicine, and is believed to promote physical, mental, and spiritual well-being. Below we will explore the key principles of Vastu Shastra and how they can be applied to create a harmonious living space.

One of the fundamental principles of Vastu Shastra is the concept of energy flow or 'prana.' The idea is that everything in the universe is made up of energy and that this energy can have a profound effect on our well-being. According to Vastu Shastra, the goal is to create a living space that allows the free flow of energy and promotes harmony between humans and nature.

One of the key elements of Vastu Shastra is the placement of objects within a living space. For example, the placement of furniture and other objects can affect the flow of energy within a room. According to Vastu Shastra, objects should be placed in such a way that they do not block the flow of energy or create any negative energy pockets. This can be achieved by arranging furniture in a way that allows for easy movement and promotes a sense of openness within the room.

Another key principle of Vastu Shastra is the use of colors in the home. According to Vastu Shastra, each color has a unique energy and can affect our emotions and well-being. For example, blue is believed to have a calming effect, while red can promote passion and energy. The use of colors in the home can be an effective way to create a harmonious living space that promotes well-being.

The orientation of a building or living space is also important in Vastu Shastra. The direction in which a building faces can affect the flow of energy and the overall well-being of its occupants. According to Vastu Shastra, buildings should be oriented in such a way that they allow for the free flow of energy and promote harmony with the natural environment. For example, buildings that face east are believed to promote health and vitality, while those that face west may be more suitable for business or commerce.

In addition to these principles, Vastu Shastra also emphasizes the importance of cleanliness and organization in the home. According to Vastu Shastra, a cluttered or dirty living space can create negative energy and disrupt the flow of energy within a room. By keeping a clean and organized home, you can promote a sense of harmony and well-being within your living space.

There are several ways to incorporate the principles of Vastu Shastra into your living space. One of the most effective ways is to use natural materials and elements in your home decor. For example, incorporating plants and natural materials like wood and stone can create a sense of harmony with nature and promote well-being. Similarly, using natural fabrics like cotton and silk can create a sense of warmth and comfort in your home.

Another way to incorporate Vastu Shastra into your home is to use lighting to create a sense of balance and harmony. According to Vastu Shastra, lighting can have a significant impact on our mood and well-being. For example, using warm, soft lighting in your living room can create a sense of comfort and relaxation, while brighter, more energizing lighting may be more suitable for a workspace.

Ayurvedic tips for a healthy kitchen

Ayurveda, the ancient Indian system of medicine, emphasizes the importance of food as medicine. Therefore, it comes as no surprise that Ayurveda places significant importance on the health of the kitchen. A healthy kitchen is not just about hygiene, but it also refers to the use of appropriate tools and cookware, storage of food, and the selection of ingredients. Below we will discuss Ayurvedic tips for a healthy kitchen that can help you promote good health and well-being.

One of the most important principles in Ayurveda is the concept of Agni, which refers to the digestive fire. According to Ayurveda, Agni plays a crucial role in the digestion and assimilation of food. Therefore, it is essential to keep the Agni strong and healthy. One of the ways to maintain a robust Agni is to cook fresh food. Freshly cooked food is easier to digest and assimilate, and it also contains a higher amount of Prana, the vital life force that is present in all living beings.

Another Ayurvedic principle for a healthy kitchen is to use appropriate cookware. Ayurveda recommends using cookware made of copper, brass, or clay. These materials are known for their heat-retaining properties and ability to distribute heat evenly, making them perfect for cooking food. Additionally, they are free of toxins, which can leach into the food during cooking. Non-stick cookware should be avoided as they are coated with chemicals that can harm the body.

Ayurveda also emphasizes the importance of the six tastes or Rasas in our food. These are sweet, sour, salty, bitter, pungent, and astringent. Each of these tastes has a specific effect on the body, and a balanced diet should include all of them. Incorporating all six tastes in our meals can help to stimulate Agni and support optimal digestion. Therefore, it is essential to use a variety of spices and herbs in cooking. Ayurvedic spices such as turmeric, cumin, coriander, ginger, and cinnamon are known for their health-promoting properties and should be a staple in every kitchen.

In Ayurveda, food is classified based on its qualities or Gunas. These Gunas refer to the physical and sensory properties of the food. The three primary Gunas are Sattva, Rajas, and Tamas. Sattvic food is pure, light, and promotes a peaceful state of mind. Rajasic food is stimulating and energizing, while Tamasic food is heavy and dulls the mind. It is recommended to eat Sattvic food as much as possible as it is the most nourishing for the body and mind. Sattvic foods include fresh fruits and vegetables, whole grains, legumes, and nuts.

Another important aspect of a healthy kitchen is storage. Ayurveda recommends storing food in a cool, dry place away from direct sunlight. This helps to preserve the vital nutrients and prevent spoilage. Food should also be stored in containers made of glass or stainless steel as they are non-toxic and do not react with the food. Plastic containers should be avoided as they can leach harmful chemicals into the food.

In Ayurveda, the concept of food combining is essential for optimal digestion. Certain food combinations can lead to indigestion, bloating, and other digestive issues. Therefore, it is recommended to avoid combining certain foods such as fruit with dairy, meat with dairy, or fruit with grains. Instead, it is best to eat foods that are compatible with each other. For example, vegetables can be eaten with grains or legumes as they complement each other.

Ayurveda for Children and Families

Ayurveda is an ancient Indian system of medicine that promotes balance and harmony within the body, mind, and spirit. It offers a holistic approach to health and wellness, and this makes it an excellent way to support the well-being of children and families.

One of the key principles of Ayurveda is that each individual is unique and has their own unique constitution, or dosha. Understanding the doshas can help parents tailor their approach to health and wellness for their children and families. The three doshas are Vata, Pitta, and Kapha, and each has its own qualities and tendencies.

Vata is characterized by movement and change, and children with a dominant Vata dosha may be creative, energetic, and imaginative. However, they may also be prone to anxiety, restlessness, and digestive issues. To support a Vata child's health, it is important to establish routines and boundaries to help them feel more grounded and secure. A Vata-pacifying diet may include warm, nourishing foods, and a consistent sleep routine can help them feel more centered and calm.

Pitta is characterized by fire and transformation, and children with a dominant Pitta dosha may be ambitious, focused, and driven. They may also be prone to irritability, impatience, and skin rashes. To support a Pitta child's health, it is important to provide them with opportunities for intellectual stimulation and creativity. A Pitta-pacifying diet may include cooling foods and avoiding spicy or fried foods. Adequate rest and relaxation can also help them maintain balance and avoid burnout.

Kapha is characterized by stability and endurance, and children with a dominant Kapha dosha may be loving, caring, and nurturing. They may also be prone to lethargy, weight gain, and congestion. To support a Kapha child's health, it is important to provide them with opportunities for physical activity and movement, as well as stimulation and variety. A Kapha-pacifying diet may include light, warming foods and spices to stimulate digestion and metabolism.

Ayurveda offers many tools and techniques to support children's health and wellness. Here are a few examples:

Abhyanga, or self-massage, can be a calming and grounding practice for children. Using warm oil, parents can massage their child's feet, hands, and scalp to promote relaxation and nourishment.

Aromatherapy can be used to support children's emotional and physical well-being. Essential oils such as lavender, chamomile, and lemon can be used in a diffuser or added to a bath to promote relaxation and calm.

Yoga and mindfulness practices can help children develop self-awareness and emotional regulation skills. Simple practices such as deep breathing and visualization can be taught to children to help them manage stress and anxiety.

Ayurveda can also be used to support families as a whole. Family routines such as meal times, bedtimes, and play times can be designed to support each individual's dosha and promote balance within the family unit. Family members can work together to create a healthy home environment that supports everyone's well-being.

Introducing Ayurveda to children

Ayurveda, a system of traditional medicine originating from India, can be incredibly beneficial for children. The principles of Ayurveda can be applied to promote physical, mental, and emotional well-being in children. Below we will explore how to introduce Ayurveda to children and incorporate its principles into their daily lives.

The first step in introducing Ayurveda to children is to make it fun and engaging. Children learn best through play, so introducing Ayurvedic principles in a playful and interactive manner is crucial. For example, parents can involve their children in cooking meals and teach them about the importance of different foods for their health. Children can also be taught about the doshas, or body types, in a way that is easy for them to understand. For example, parents can relate Vata dosha to the wind, Pitta dosha to the fire, and Kapha dosha to the earth. This helps children to remember and understand the doshas.

Incorporating Ayurvedic practices into children's daily routines can also be beneficial. A morning routine that includes tongue scraping and oil pulling can help remove toxins and promote oral hygiene. Parents can also encourage their children to spend time outdoors in nature, which is grounding and soothing for the nervous system. Additionally, practicing meditation or yoga together can be a great way to teach children how to manage stress and emotions.

Ayurveda also offers various herbal remedies that can be used for common ailments in children. For example, ginger tea can be used to relieve nausea and soothe the digestive system, while chamomile tea can help calm the mind and promote restful sleep. Turmeric can be used to reduce inflammation, and honey can be used to soothe sore throats.

It is important to note that Ayurvedic remedies should be used under the guidance of a qualified Ayurvedic practitioner or healthcare provider. Children have developing bodies, and certain herbs and remedies may not be appropriate for their age or health condition.

Ayurveda also emphasizes the importance of seasonal living. Children can be taught about the changing seasons and how to adjust their lifestyles accordingly. For example, in the winter, children can be encouraged to eat warming foods like soups and stews, while in the summer, they can be encouraged to eat cooling foods like salads and fruits.

In addition to physical health, Ayurveda also promotes emotional well-being. Children can be taught about the importance of emotional balance and how to manage their emotions in a healthy way. For example, parents can teach their children about the concept of mindfulness and encourage them to practice it daily. This can involve simple practices like taking a few deep breaths or practicing gratitude.

Ayurveda also emphasizes the importance of self-care. Children can be taught about the importance of taking care of their bodies and minds. For example, parents can encourage their children to take breaks from technology and spend time doing activities that promote relaxation and creativity. This can include activities like reading, drawing, or spending time in nature.

Ayurvedic remedies for common childhood ailments

Ayurveda, the ancient Indian system of medicine, has been used for thousands of years to treat a wide range of ailments, including those that commonly afflict children. Ayurvedic remedies are safe, natural, and effective, and can be used to address a variety of childhood health issues, from minor complaints like coughs and colds to more serious conditions like asthma and allergies. Below we will explore some of the most effective Ayurvedic remedies for common childhood ailments.

1. Coughs and Colds: One of the most common ailments that affects children is the cough and cold. To treat these conditions, Ayurveda recommends the use of herbs like ginger, turmeric, and honey. These ingredients have natural anti-inflammatory and antibacterial properties that can help soothe the throat and reduce congestion. Parents can give children a mixture of honey and ginger juice to alleviate the symptoms of cough and cold. Turmeric mixed with milk is also a popular remedy to treat coughs and colds.

2. Digestive Problems: Children often suffer from digestive problems such as constipation, diarrhea, and stomachache. Ayurveda recommends the use of digestive herbs like ginger, fennel, and coriander to alleviate these issues. Fennel and coriander seeds can be boiled in water to make a tea that can be given to children to improve digestion and relieve stomachache. Ginger can be added to food or tea to help with constipation and other digestive issues.

3. Skin Problems: Children are prone to skin problems like eczema, rashes, and acne. Ayurvedic remedies for these conditions include the use of herbs like neem and turmeric. Neem has antibacterial and antifungal properties that can help clear up skin infections, while turmeric has anti-inflammatory properties that can reduce redness and swelling. A paste made from neem leaves and turmeric can be applied to the affected area to treat skin problems in children.

4. Allergies: Many children suffer from allergies, particularly those related to pollen, dust, and animal dander. Ayurveda recommends the use of herbs like turmeric, licorice, and ashwagandha to alleviate the symptoms of allergies. Turmeric can be added to milk or taken as a supplement to help reduce inflammation, while licorice and ashwagandha can help strengthen the immune system.

5. Asthma: Asthma is a chronic respiratory condition that affects many children. Ayurvedic remedies for asthma include the use of herbs like ginger, black pepper, and honey. These ingredients can help reduce inflammation in the airways and make it easier for children to breathe. A mixture of honey and black pepper can be given to children to alleviate asthma symptoms, while ginger tea can be used as a natural bronchodilator.

In addition to these specific remedies, Ayurveda recommends a number of general practices that can help keep children healthy and prevent illness. These include:

6. Maintaining a healthy diet: Ayurveda recommends a balanced diet that includes a variety of fruits, vegetables, whole grains, and lean proteins. Avoiding processed foods, sugary snacks, and fried foods can help keep children healthy and reduce the risk of illness.

7. Getting enough sleep: Children need plenty of rest to stay healthy and maintain their energy levels. Ayurveda recommends a regular sleep schedule and a calming bedtime routine to help children fall asleep and stay asleep throughout the night.

8. Staying active: Regular exercise is important for children's physical and mental health. Ayurveda recommends activities like yoga, dance, and sports to keep children active and engaged.

9. Managing stress: Stress can have a negative impact on children's health, both physical and mental. Ayurveda recommends practices like meditation

Building a healthy family lifestyle with Ayurveda

Ayurveda is an ancient system of medicine that originated in India thousands of years ago. It is a holistic approach that emphasizes the importance of maintaining balance between the mind, body, and spirit. Ayurveda offers a variety of practices and remedies that can be used to promote a healthy family lifestyle.

One of the primary principles of Ayurveda is the concept of doshas. There are three doshas - Vata, Pitta, and Kapha - that are present in all individuals in varying degrees. Each dosha has unique characteristics and influences different aspects of the mind and body. By understanding the dominant dosha of each family member, Ayurveda can help tailor practices and remedies that support optimal health.

A healthy family lifestyle begins with nutrition. Ayurveda recommends a diet that is balanced and nourishing for each individual's dosha. A Vata-dominant individual, for example, may benefit from warm, grounding foods such as root vegetables and whole grains. A Pitta-dominant individual may thrive on cooling, refreshing foods such as cucumbers and leafy greens. And a Kapha-dominant individual may benefit from stimulating, light foods such as spicy peppers and bitter greens.

In addition to a balanced diet, Ayurveda recommends a daily routine that supports optimal health. This routine, known as dinacharya, may include practices such as meditation, yoga, and self-massage. By establishing a consistent daily routine, families can create a sense of stability and balance that supports overall health and well-being.

Ayurveda also offers a variety of remedies for common childhood ailments. For example, ginger and honey tea can be used to soothe a sore throat, while chamomile tea can help promote calm and relaxation. Turmeric, a powerful anti-inflammatory herb, can be used to support healthy digestion and reduce inflammation throughout the body.

In addition to dietary and lifestyle practices, Ayurveda also emphasizes the importance of creating a healthy living environment. This includes maintaining a clean and organized home, using non-toxic cleaning products, and incorporating natural elements such as plants and fresh air.

Ayurveda can also be used to support mental and emotional health within the family. For example, parents may benefit from practices such as meditation and pranayama (breathing exercises) to help reduce stress and promote relaxation. Children can also benefit from mindfulness practices, such as guided meditation and deep breathing exercises, to help promote focus and calm.

Another key aspect of Ayurvedic family health is maintaining healthy relationships. This includes cultivating a sense of connection and communication within the family, as well as practicing forgiveness and compassion. By fostering a sense of love and understanding within the family unit, individuals can support each other in maintaining optimal health and well-being.

Ayurvedic Travel and Wellness Retreats

Ayurveda, the ancient Indian system of medicine, offers a holistic approach to health and wellness that emphasizes the balance between the body, mind, and spirit. While Ayurvedic principles can be integrated into everyday life at home, there are also many opportunities for immersive experiences through Ayurvedic travel and wellness retreats.

Ayurvedic travel and wellness retreats offer a chance to escape from the stress of daily life and focus on rejuvenation and healing through Ayurvedic practices. These retreats can be found around the world, from India to Europe to the United States, and offer a range of programs and accommodations to fit individual needs and preferences.

One of the key aspects of Ayurvedic travel and wellness retreats is the emphasis on personalized care. Ayurvedic practitioners use a comprehensive approach to assess each individual's unique constitution or dosha and create customized treatment plans tailored to their specific needs. This can include herbal remedies, massage therapies, dietary recommendations, and meditation and yoga practices.

Many Ayurvedic travel and wellness retreats also offer classes and workshops to help participants learn more about Ayurvedic principles and practices. This can include cooking classes to learn how to prepare Ayurvedic meals, yoga classes to promote physical and mental well-being, and meditation classes to help reduce stress and anxiety.

In addition to personalized care and educational opportunities, Ayurvedic travel and wellness retreats often provide a tranquil and serene environment to promote relaxation and rejuvenation. This can include natural surroundings such as mountains or beaches, as well as spa facilities and amenities such as hot springs or saunas.

Ayurvedic travel and wellness retreats can be beneficial for individuals seeking relief from specific health conditions, as well as for those who simply want to focus on maintaining overall health and wellness. Some of the health conditions that Ayurvedic travel and wellness retreats may address include digestive issues, stress and anxiety, insomnia, and skin disorders.

For those interested in Ayurvedic travel and wellness retreats, it is important to research and choose a reputable and experienced provider. It is also important to communicate any health conditions or concerns with the retreat staff and to follow any recommendations or guidelines provided to ensure a safe and beneficial experience.

Tips for maintaining Ayurvedic balance while traveling

Ayurveda, the ancient Indian system of medicine, emphasizes the importance of maintaining balance and harmony within the body and mind. This balance is essential for optimal health and well-being. However, travel can disrupt this balance, leading to imbalances in the doshas, which are the energies that govern our body and mind.

Fortunately, there are several Ayurvedic tips and practices that can help maintain balance and promote wellness while traveling.

1. Follow a daily routine: Ayurveda places great importance on following a daily routine, as it helps to maintain balance and stability in the body and mind. Even when traveling, it is important to establish a routine that includes waking up and going to bed at the same time every day, eating meals at regular intervals, and taking time to relax and recharge.

2. Stay hydrated: Travel can be dehydrating, and dehydration can lead to imbalances in the doshas. It is important to drink plenty of water and other hydrating fluids, such as coconut water or herbal tea, throughout the day.

3. Choose the right foods: The foods we eat have a direct impact on our doshas. While traveling, it is important to choose foods that are nourishing, easy to digest, and appropriate for your dosha. This may include fresh fruits and vegetables, whole grains, lean protein, and healthy fats.

4. Practice gentle yoga and meditation: Yoga and meditation are powerful tools for maintaining balance and reducing stress. Even a few minutes of deep breathing, gentle stretching, or meditation can help to calm the mind and promote relaxation.

5. Use essential oils: Essential oils can be used to balance the doshas and promote wellness while traveling. Lavender, for example, is known for its calming properties, while peppermint can help to soothe digestion.

6. Get enough sleep: Adequate sleep is essential for maintaining balance and promoting wellness. When traveling, it can be tempting to stay up late and wake up early to make the most of your trip. However, it is important to prioritize sleep and make sure you are getting enough rest each night.

7. Avoid excessive stimulation: Travel can be overwhelming, with new sights, sounds, and experiences at every turn. While it is important to explore and enjoy your destination, it is also important to take breaks and avoid excessive stimulation. This may include taking a quiet walk in nature, reading a book, or simply sitting and taking in the surroundings.

8. Take time to rest and recharge: Travel can be exciting, but it can also be exhausting. It is important to take time to rest and recharge, whether that means taking a nap, enjoying a massage, or simply sitting and doing nothing for a few minutes.

By following these Ayurvedic tips and practices, you can maintain balance and promote wellness while traveling. Whether you are on a business trip, a family vacation, or a solo adventure, these simple strategies can help you feel your best and make the most of your travel experience.

Ayurvedic wellness retreats around the world

Ayurvedic wellness retreats have become increasingly popular in recent years as people seek to rejuvenate their mind, body, and spirit through traditional Ayurvedic practices. These retreats offer an opportunity to disconnect from the stress of daily life and immerse oneself in a healing environment that promotes holistic health and wellness. Here, we will explore some of the best Ayurvedic wellness retreats around the world.

Kairali Ayurvedic Healing Village, India

Located in the southern Indian state of Kerala, Kairali Ayurvedic Healing Village is a world-renowned Ayurvedic wellness center. This lush resort is situated on 50 acres of verdant land and offers a wide range of Ayurvedic treatments, including Panchakarma therapy, massages, and yoga classes. Kairali also has an organic farm and serves delicious vegetarian meals prepared according to Ayurvedic principles.

Shanti Maurice Resort & Spa, Mauritius

Shanti Maurice Resort & Spa in Mauritius is an idyllic beachfront property that offers a unique blend of Ayurveda and luxury. The resort features a dedicated Ayurvedic spa that offers a range of treatments, including Abhyanga, Shirodhara, and Nasyam. The Ayurvedic menu at Shanti Maurice's restaurant uses local, organic ingredients and is tailored to individual Doshas.

Vana, India

Vana is a luxurious Ayurvedic wellness retreat in Dehradun, India. The retreat offers a range of Ayurvedic treatments, including Abhyanga, Kizhi, and Pizhichil, as well as personalized yoga and meditation programs. Vana also features an Ayurvedic pharmacy, a library, and organic gardens that provide fresh produce for the restaurant.

Hamsa Ayurveda & Yoga Shala, Sri Lanka

Hamsa Ayurveda & Yoga Shala is a charming Ayurvedic retreat in the southern Sri Lankan town of Ahangama. The retreat offers a variety of Ayurvedic treatments, including Abhyanga, Shirodhara, and Pinda Sweda. Hamsa also has a beautiful yoga shala overlooking the ocean and serves organic vegetarian meals.

Ananda in the Himalayas, India

Ananda in the Himalayas is a luxurious Ayurvedic wellness retreat in the foothills of the Himalayas. The retreat offers a range of Ayurvedic treatments, including Panchakarma therapy, massages, and yoga classes. Ananda's restaurant serves organic vegetarian meals that are tailored to individual Doshas.

COMO Shambhala Estate, Bali

COMO Shambhala Estate is a wellness retreat in the heart of Bali that offers a range of Ayurvedic treatments, including Abhyanga, Shirodhara, and Nasyam. The retreat also features a beautiful yoga pavilion and offers customized wellness programs that combine Ayurveda, yoga, and other healing modalities. The restaurant serves healthy, organic cuisine that is tailored to individual needs.

Santani Wellness Resort & Spa, Sri Lanka

Santani Wellness Resort & Spa is a beautiful Ayurvedic retreat nestled in the hills of Sri Lanka. The retreat offers a range of Ayurvedic treatments, including Panchakarma therapy, massages, and yoga classes. Santani's restaurant serves delicious, organic cuisine that is tailored to individual Doshas.

Creating your own Ayurvedic retreat experience at home

Ayurveda is a holistic healing system that emphasizes balance and harmony between the mind, body, and spirit. This ancient Indian practice provides a wide range of tools and practices that can be utilized to create a wellness retreat experience at home. While there are many Ayurvedic retreat centers around the world that offer various treatments and therapies, there are also many simple practices that can be incorporated into daily life to create a personalized Ayurvedic retreat experience.

The first step in creating an Ayurvedic retreat experience at home is to establish a daily routine or dinacharya. This routine should include practices such as waking up early, drinking warm water with lemon, practicing meditation or yoga, and having a healthy breakfast. Ayurveda emphasizes the importance of consistency and routine in maintaining balance and harmony, so sticking to a daily routine is key to creating an Ayurvedic lifestyle.

Another important aspect of an Ayurvedic retreat experience is incorporating healthy and nourishing foods into one's diet. Ayurveda places a strong emphasis on eating whole, seasonal foods that are fresh and locally sourced. Foods that are easy to digest and provide nourishment to the body, such as fresh fruits and vegetables, whole grains, and healthy fats, should be prioritized. Ayurveda also recommends avoiding processed foods, refined sugars, and artificial ingredients.

In addition to nourishing foods, Ayurveda also provides a wide range of herbs and spices that can be used for healing and wellness. Herbs such as ashwagandha, turmeric, and triphala have been used for centuries to support overall health and wellbeing. These herbs can be added to meals or consumed in supplement form to support digestion, boost immunity, and promote relaxation.

Ayurveda also places a strong emphasis on self-care practices, such as abhyanga or self-massage, which involves massaging the body with warm oil to promote relaxation and circulation. This practice can be easily incorporated into a home Ayurvedic retreat experience by setting aside time each day to practice self-massage.

In addition to self-massage, other self-care practices that can be incorporated into an Ayurvedic retreat experience include aromatherapy, pranayama or breathing exercises, and journaling. Aromatherapy involves using essential oils to promote relaxation and support overall wellbeing. Pranayama involves focusing on the breath to calm the mind and promote relaxation. Journaling can be a helpful practice for processing emotions and reflecting on one's thoughts and experiences.

Lastly, incorporating movement and exercise into an Ayurvedic retreat experience is important for promoting physical and mental wellbeing. Yoga and other forms of gentle movement, such as walking or swimming, can be helpful for reducing stress, improving circulation, and promoting relaxation.

In addition to these practices, creating a peaceful and calming environment can also contribute to an Ayurvedic retreat experience at home. This can be achieved through practices such as decluttering, using calming colors and lighting, and incorporating natural elements such as plants or crystals.

Resources for Learning More about Ayurveda

Ayurveda, the traditional Indian system of medicine, has been gaining popularity in recent years as people seek holistic approaches to health and wellness. Whether you are new to Ayurveda or are already familiar with its principles, there are many resources available to help you deepen your understanding and integrate Ayurvedic practices into your life.

1. Books are a great place to start when learning about Ayurveda. There are many books on the topic, ranging from introductions to in-depth manuals on specific topics. Some popular options include "The Complete Book of Ayurvedic Home Remedies" by Vasant Lad, "Ayurveda: The Science of Self-Healing" by Dr. Vasant Lad, and "The Everyday Ayurveda Cookbook" by Kate O'Donnell. These books offer a wealth of information on Ayurvedic principles, remedies, and practices.

In addition to books, there are many online resources available for learning about Ayurveda. Websites such as Banyan Botanicals, The Ayurveda Experience, and Yoga Journal offer articles, videos, and courses on Ayurvedic topics. These resources are a great way to learn about Ayurveda from the comfort of your own home.

If you are interested in studying Ayurveda in depth, there are many schools and training programs available. Some popular options include the Ayurvedic Institute in Albuquerque, New Mexico, the California College of Ayurveda, and the Kripalu School of Ayurveda in Massachusetts. These programs offer a variety of courses and certifications for those interested in becoming Ayurvedic practitioners.

Ayurvedic practitioners and clinics can also be a valuable resource for learning about Ayurveda. A qualified practitioner can provide personalized guidance on Ayurvedic practices and remedies based on your unique constitution and health concerns. Many practitioners also offer workshops and classes to help individuals learn more about Ayurvedic principles and practices.

Finally, Ayurvedic products can be a helpful resource for incorporating Ayurvedic practices into your daily routine. Products such as herbal supplements, oils, and skincare products are available from a variety of sources. However, it is important to ensure that you are purchasing high-quality, authentic Ayurvedic products from reputable sources.

Ayurvedic schools and certification programs

Ayurveda, the ancient Indian system of medicine, has gained popularity in recent years as a holistic approach to wellness. With its focus on balance and individualization, Ayurveda offers a unique perspective on health and healing that is not found in Western medicine. For those interested in deepening their knowledge of Ayurveda, there are a variety of schools and certification programs available. Below we will explore some of the top Ayurvedic schools and certification programs and what they offer to students.

One of the most well-known Ayurvedic schools is the California College of Ayurveda. Founded in 1995, the college offers a range of programs from introductory workshops to full professional certification. Their programs are designed to be accessible to students with different backgrounds and interests, including healthcare professionals, yoga teachers, and those looking to deepen their personal understanding of Ayurveda. The college has a strong emphasis on practical learning and offers hands-on clinical experience to students in addition to classroom instruction.

Another prominent Ayurvedic school is the Ayurvedic Institute, founded by Dr. Vasant Lad in 1984. The institute offers a range of programs, including a one-year Ayurvedic Studies Program and a three-year Professional Ayurvedic Studies Program. In addition to their standard programs, the institute also offers specialized courses in areas such as pulse diagnosis, herbal formulation, and Panchakarma (an Ayurvedic detoxification treatment). The institute is known for its strong focus on Ayurvedic philosophy and spirituality, making it an attractive option for those interested in a more holistic approach to wellness.

The Mount Madonna Institute, located in California, offers a Master of Arts in Ayurveda program that is one of the most comprehensive Ayurvedic programs available. The program is designed for students who want to become Ayurvedic practitioners and offers a deep dive into the theory, philosophy, and practice of Ayurveda. In addition to classroom instruction, students receive hands-on clinical experience through internships at the Mount Madonna Center, a yoga and Ayurvedic retreat center affiliated with the institute.

For those interested in online learning, the Kripalu School of Ayurveda offers a range of programs and courses that can be taken from anywhere in the world. The school's flagship program is a 650-hour Ayurvedic Health Counselor Certification Program, which is designed for those who want to integrate Ayurveda into their existing healthcare practice or offer Ayurvedic consultations as a standalone service. The program includes online coursework, live webinars, and a five-day immersion at the Kripalu Center for Yoga & Health in Massachusetts.

The Ayurvedic Studies Program at the New York Open Center is another option for those interested in online learning. The program is designed to provide a comprehensive understanding of Ayurveda from both a theoretical and practical perspective. Students receive instruction from experienced Ayurvedic practitioners and have the opportunity to participate in supervised clinical internships. The program can be taken in-person or online, making it a flexible option for students with different schedules and locations.

Finally, for those looking for a more immersive Ayurvedic experience, there are a variety of Ayurvedic retreats and workshops available around the world. Many of these retreats offer the opportunity to learn about Ayurveda in a hands-on, experiential way while also enjoying the benefits of Ayurvedic treatments and practices. Examples of Ayurvedic retreats include the Shankara Ayurveda Spa in Kerala, India, and the Shakti Ayurveda School in British Columbia, Canada.

Books, websites, and online courses

Ayurveda, an ancient system of health and healing, has been gaining popularity in recent years as people look for alternative and holistic approaches to wellness. As interest in Ayurveda grows, so does the availability of resources for learning more about this powerful system. Below we will explore some of the best books, websites, and online courses for those interested in deepening their understanding of Ayurveda.

Books:

1. There are countless books available on Ayurveda, but some stand out as particularly informative and accessible to beginners. One classic text is "The Complete Book of Ayurvedic Home Remedies" by Dr. Vasant Lad. This book covers a wide range of topics, from basic principles of Ayurveda to remedies for specific health issues. Another highly recommended book is "Ayurveda: The Science of Self-Healing" by Dr. Vasant Lad, which provides a clear and concise introduction to Ayurvedic principles and practices.

2. For those interested in diving deeper into Ayurvedic philosophy and spirituality, "The Ayurveda Way: 108 Practices from the World's Oldest Healing System for Better Sleep, Less Stress, Optimal Digestion, and More" by Ananta Ripa Ajmera is an excellent resource. This book explores Ayurvedic principles and practices for mind-body balance and includes practical tips for incorporating these practices into daily life.

Websites:

The internet is an excellent resource for learning more about Ayurveda. One website that stands out is Banyan Botanicals, which offers a wealth of information on Ayurvedic principles and practices, as well as high-quality Ayurvedic products. The site includes a blog with informative articles on a wide range of Ayurvedic topics, and they also offer a free dosha quiz to help visitors determine their unique Ayurvedic constitution.

Another excellent website is the Ayurvedic Institute, founded by Dr. Vasant Lad. This site offers information on Ayurvedic education, as well as online courses and resources for those interested in deepening their understanding of Ayurvedic philosophy and practices.

Online Courses:

For those looking for a more structured and immersive learning experience, there are a variety of online courses available on Ayurveda. The Ayurvedic Institute offers several online courses, including an Introduction to Ayurveda course and an Ayurvedic Health Counselor program. The California College of Ayurveda also offers online courses, including a Professional Ayurvedic Continuing Education program and an Ayurvedic Health Practitioner program.

Another excellent resource is the Chopra Center, founded by Drs. Deepak Chopra and David Simon. The center offers a variety of online courses, including an Ayurvedic Wellness Counselor program and an Ayurvedic Cooking course.

Finding an Ayurvedic practitioner and community

Ayurveda is an ancient Indian system of holistic medicine that emphasizes the interconnectedness of the mind, body, and spirit. Ayurvedic practitioners use a range of treatments and therapies, including herbal remedies, dietary changes, and lifestyle modifications, to help their patients achieve optimal health and well-being. If you are interested in exploring the benefits of Ayurveda for yourself, it can be helpful to seek out a qualified Ayurvedic practitioner and join an Ayurvedic community. Below we will discuss some tips for finding an Ayurvedic practitioner and community that can support your health and wellness journey.

One way to find an Ayurvedic practitioner is to ask for recommendations from friends, family members, or healthcare providers who have experience with Ayurveda. They may be able to refer you to a reputable practitioner in your area. Alternatively, you can search online for Ayurvedic practitioners in your area. There are many directories and databases that list Ayurvedic practitioners, such as the National Ayurvedic Medical Association and the Ayurvedic Institute.

When choosing an Ayurvedic practitioner, it is important to look for someone who has received adequate training and certification. In the United States, the National Ayurvedic Medical Association provides a certification program for Ayurvedic practitioners, and many states also have licensing requirements. It is also important to choose a practitioner who has experience treating your specific health concerns or conditions.

Once you have found an Ayurvedic practitioner, you may also want to consider joining an Ayurvedic community. This can provide a supportive environment for learning more about Ayurveda and practicing its principles in your daily life. There are many Ayurvedic communities online, such as forums and social media groups, where you can connect with other people who share your interest in Ayurveda. You can also search for local Ayurvedic groups and workshops in your area.

1. In addition to finding an Ayurvedic practitioner and community, there are also many resources available to help you learn more about Ayurveda on your own. There are numerous books on Ayurveda written for both beginners and advanced practitioners, such as "The Complete Book of Ayurvedic Home Remedies" by Dr. Vasant Lad and "Ayurveda: The Science of Self-Healing" by Dr. Vasant Lad. There are also many online courses and workshops that can provide in-depth instruction on Ayurvedic principles and practices.

Reflecting on your Ayurvedic journey

Ayurveda is an ancient Indian system of holistic health that has gained popularity around the world in recent years. This approach to health and wellness is based on the belief that each person is a unique combination of three doshas, or energies, that determine their physical, mental, and emotional characteristics. By understanding one's dosha and making lifestyle choices that support it, one can achieve optimal health and well-being.

Embarking on an Ayurvedic journey can be a transformative experience that helps one connect with their body, mind, and spirit. However, it's important to approach this journey with an open mind and a willingness to make changes to one's lifestyle. Below we will reflect on some important aspects of the Ayurvedic journey, including self-awareness, self-care, and community.

Self-awareness is a key component of the Ayurvedic journey. This means taking the time to observe and understand one's own body, mind, and emotions. It involves paying attention to the signals that the body is sending, such as hunger, fatigue, and pain, and making choices that support overall health and well-being. Self-awareness also involves understanding one's dosha and the unique characteristics that it brings.

One important aspect of self-awareness in Ayurveda is recognizing the impact of food on the body. Food is considered a powerful medicine in Ayurveda, and making the right choices can have a significant impact on overall health. This includes choosing foods that are appropriate for one's dosha and avoiding foods that are not. It also means taking the time to eat mindfully, paying attention to the flavors, textures, and aromas of the food and savoring each bite.

Another key aspect of the Ayurvedic journey is self-care. This involves making choices that support physical, mental, and emotional health. This includes developing a daily routine that supports one's dosha, such as choosing the right type of exercise and getting enough sleep. Self-care also means taking time for relaxation and stress reduction, such as through meditation, yoga, or other practices.

Ayurveda also emphasizes the importance of community in the journey towards optimal health and well-being. Finding a supportive community of like-minded individuals can be an important part of this journey. This includes seeking out Ayurvedic practitioners who can provide guidance and support, as well as connecting with others who share a similar interest in Ayurveda.

Another important aspect of community in Ayurveda is the idea of seva, or service. This involves finding ways to give back to one's community and help others on their own journey towards health and wellness. This might involve volunteering at a local community center, teaching others about Ayurveda, or sharing healthy recipes and lifestyle tips with friends and family.

Cultivating a lifelong commitment to Ayurvedic principles

Ayurveda, a traditional Indian system of medicine, offers a holistic approach to health and wellness that has been practiced for thousands of years. Its principles emphasize the importance of balancing the body, mind, and spirit to achieve optimal health and prevent disease. By incorporating Ayurvedic principles into your daily routine and lifestyle, you can cultivate a lifelong commitment to wellness that will benefit you in countless ways.

1. One of the key tenets of Ayurveda is the recognition that each individual is unique and requires personalized care. This is based on the concept of the doshas, or the three energetic forces that govern the body and mind: Vata, Pitta, and Kapha. Each individual has a unique combination of these doshas, which determines their physical and mental characteristics, as well as their susceptibility to certain imbalances and health conditions.

To cultivate a lifelong commitment to Ayurvedic principles, it is important to understand your own dosha constitution and how to maintain balance. You can start by consulting with an Ayurvedic practitioner or taking an online quiz to determine your dosha type. Once you know your dosha, you can begin to make dietary and lifestyle choices that support your unique needs.

One of the most important ways to maintain balance is through diet. Ayurveda recommends eating whole, fresh, and seasonal foods that are appropriate for your dosha type. For example, Vata types may benefit from warm, grounding foods such as root vegetables, while Pitta types may benefit from cooling, hydrating foods such as cucumbers and watermelon. Kapha types may benefit from lighter, spicier foods to stimulate their metabolism.

In addition to diet, Ayurveda emphasizes the importance of daily self-care practices to maintain balance. This includes practices such as oil massage (abhyanga), meditation, yoga, and pranayama (breathing exercises). These practices help to calm the mind, reduce stress, and promote overall well-being.

Another important aspect of Ayurvedic lifestyle is sleep hygiene. Adequate sleep is essential for overall health and wellness, and Ayurveda recommends going to bed early and rising early to align with the natural rhythms of the day. It also recommends avoiding screens and other stimulating activities before bedtime, and creating a relaxing sleep environment.

Finally, cultivating a lifelong commitment to Ayurvedic principles means incorporating them into your daily life and making them a part of your routine. This may include setting aside time for self-care practices, meal planning and preparation, and creating a supportive environment in your home and workplace. It may also involve seeking out community support, such as joining an Ayurvedic health group or attending retreats and workshops.

Sharing the benefits of Ayurveda with others

Ayurveda is a powerful system of medicine that has been used for thousands of years in India and is becoming increasingly popular worldwide. While Ayurveda offers many benefits to those who practice it, it can also be a challenge to introduce it to others. However, sharing the benefits of Ayurveda with others is important because it can improve their overall health and well-being.

One way to share the benefits of Ayurveda is to educate others about the principles of Ayurveda. This includes teaching them about the three doshas (Vata, Pitta, and Kapha) and how they influence our physical, mental, and emotional health. You can explain how to determine one's dosha and how to balance it through diet, lifestyle, and herbal remedies.

Another way to share Ayurveda with others is to encourage them to try Ayurvedic practices for themselves. This can include introducing them to simple practices such as daily self-massage (abhyanga), tongue scraping, or oil pulling. You can also encourage them to attend an Ayurvedic cooking class or to try a yoga or meditation class that incorporates Ayurvedic principles.

It's important to remember that Ayurveda is not a one-size-fits-all approach, and what works for one person may not work for another. Encouraging others to work with a qualified Ayurvedic practitioner can help them get personalized recommendations that will be most effective for their individual needs.

When sharing Ayurveda with others, it's important to approach the topic with an open and non-judgmental mindset. Many people may be unfamiliar with Ayurveda and may not understand its benefits. It's important to explain the principles in a clear and concise manner, without overwhelming them with too much information at once.

One effective way to introduce Ayurveda to others is to lead by example. By incorporating Ayurvedic practices into your own life and sharing your experiences with others, you can inspire them to try Ayurveda for themselves. This can include sharing simple recipes, discussing the benefits of a daily routine, or talking about how Ayurveda has improved your own health.

Finally, it's important to keep in mind that Ayurveda is a holistic approach to health and well-being. Encouraging others to incorporate Ayurvedic principles into their lives is not just about improving their physical health, but also their mental and emotional health. This includes promoting self-care, stress reduction, and mindfulness practices.

Have Questions / Comments?

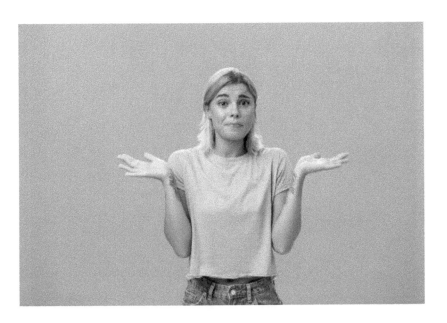

This book was designed to cover as much as possible but I know I have probably missed something, or some new amazing discovery that has just come out.

If you notice something missing or have a question that I failed to answer, please get in touch and let me know. If I can, I will email you an answer and also update the book so others can also benefit from it.

Thanks For Being Awesome :)

Submit Your Questions / Comments At:

https://xspurts.com/posts/questions

---

1. https://xspurts.com/posts/questions

Get Another Book Free

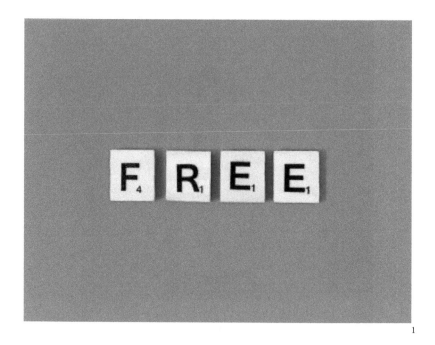

We love writing and have produced a huge number of books.

For being one of our amazing readers, we would love to offer you another book we have created, 100% free.

To claim this limited time special offer, simply go to the site below and enter your name and email address.

You will then receive one of my great books, direct to your email account, 100% free!

https://xspurts.com/posts/free-book-offer

---

1. https://xspurts.com/posts/free-book-offer

Also by Mei Lin Zhang